CW00888947

Welcome to my World

Gellespi Donks

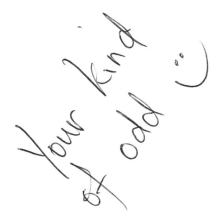

chipmunkapublishing
the mental health publisher

Gellespi Donks

Published by
Chipmunkapublishing
PO Box 6872
Brentwood
Essex CM13 1ZT
United Kingdom

http://www.chipmunkapublishing.com

Chipmunkapublishing gratefully acknowledge the support of Arts Council England.

2

**For my dad,
"just a smile away"**

Gellespi Donks

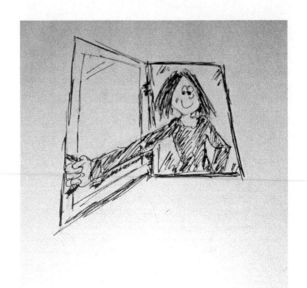

Welcome to My World

Authors note

My big 'thank yous' are to my family and friends, without you I would be empty. For Patti, you kept me dry when it rained so hard and for Jane, who unlocked the world that sits outside of mine. Fee and Paul you know too much about full stops and Tash, nice colouring in.

Finally always my perfect day dream…another time, another place.

In my world every thing is simple, I don't complicate things.
There is a 'right' and a 'wrong', a good and a bad.
In my world the flowers, the trees and the sun make up the rainbow.
The laughter, the smiles and the people I love make the memories that fill it with colour.
There is always a pot full up of dreams
Chasing rainbows is fun. It's simple and it is who I am…
Welcome to my world.

Gellespi Donks

Chapter One

I was sitting, looking out of the window in a coffee house. I'm calling it that to provide a slightly more up market vision and something just a little bit cosmopolitan, because really that's how I felt that day. I'd had a succession of small but poignant achievements. These, I felt, qualified me to be, dare I say it, confident. Firstly I had walked past my mirror at home and impressed by my choice of clothes, ones that matched, I gave the girl that stared back a wink. This was success number one. Secondly I hadn't waved at anyone I didn't know as I drove into the town. A positive result I felt, as ordinarily I received so many toots and waves not always very traditional in waving technique. More gestures I suppose you would class them as. I strolled into the coffee house (see what I'm doing there, drawing you in with that cosmopolitan touch again). I ordered from the counter a café latte (slightly continental I felt) and I did this in only the 4 syllables required. I have been known to add a few extra whilst in a less confident state and in doing this I would usually receive a reply suited perhaps more for someone hard of hearing. There would also be an uncomfortable silence and lots of awkward smiling which really made me relax!!

So here I was 3 successful achievements and then I saw it….the window seat or should I say the window bar stool. Often avoided for fear of the whole mounting procedure I felt strong and able and so I approached. I climbed (ok so there was some apprehension) up those daunting side steps to reach my destination….the top of the stool. I'd nailed it. This much sought after seat was my throne for the morning. No one was getting near this baby for the duration of my latte and I owned that place. This cosmopolitan girl was at her station. The dismount.....well that was going to be a whole new challenge...Clearly I have digressed from my story but the stool thing.....got to be worth a mention.

Somebody had asked me recently what motivates me. It was an easy to answer question but not so simple to find the words to explain. So I'm sat staring out of the window in a somewhat Enya style video promo and I start to think (its ok I keep that exercise to a minimum) how do you find the words that help someone to understand.... So I'm gazing, and I'm thinking and then there she was.....the one that all try to avoid. The one that has tripped into the coffee house, bags aplenty, comedy waved at everyone and was now blocking my picturesque view. The day I got the best seat in the house I got the friendly stranger nobody wants to talk to perch her very cushioned arse next to me. I looked up...my fault entirely. The neon sign that reads 'all eccentric, unusual and sometimes scary people approach, I welcome you', was glowing invitingly above me. I had forgotten in my confident mirage to turn it off. And so I had company. "Please don't talk, please don't, I won't answer, I'll look away...." my thoughts were so loud I hoped she could hear them. Alas it was the Bart Simpson ear muffs that muffled my plea and she spoke and worse still.....I answered.

I was well practiced at unusual intros....my friend chip, I'd called him that due to his uncanny likeness to the Chippendales (oh how I silently laughed) when he introduced me to his wife she said "hi I'm Fiona and I have IBS,". At the time I was not well practiced in the now very abbreviated world and so I enquired further. "IBS?" "Irritable bowel syndrome" she stated.... Boy he'd bagged a good'un! "Hi" I'd replied. "My sister can say her whole name, address and postcode in a burp!"

Welcome to My World

We never really had a lot in common after that initial chat.

Again I have been sidetracked; I will try to keep to my story. So Miss 'lardy bloater' in front of me began. I'm guessing she was around 17 maybe 18 and that the chubby look was not from an extensive course of steroids. My friend had the unfortunate experience of steroid fat person side effect and when I saw her I was scared as it had really looked like her cheeks had eaten her eyes. So she began...polite intros and a welfare check. Intriguing but we have all fallen victim to the 'how are you' oops no time for a reply type conversation. She seemed keen to engage me with chat and as my latte cosmopolitan experience slipped reluctantly away I listened....first in a fixed 'I'm not interested' way.

"I'm in town today, just been to court." Lardy spoke.

My lip did a bit of a slightly Elvis curl. I did not want to be sitting in the coffee house next to someone who thought their sofa was best placed in the front garden along with countless other electrical items. Undeterred by the lip thing she continued. "I got off with a ban."

My thoughts of "don't ask what for, I am wondering though but don't ask" were broken by her reply "well that's the thing"
I looked up. The Bart Simpson earmuffs were off.... oh my god she'd heard me!

And so she continued. "I was I bit of a rebel at school" (ok I thought, me too, all be it with Clarks shoes, a blazer and a purdey haircut my mother insisted on tonging into place daily, don't doubt it I have the scars on each ear.) She told me that things had gone a bit pear shaped at her school.

Wasn't that what school was all about I thought? Written in the curriculum to prepare kids for the grown up world? I threw her a very unsympathetic Elvis snarl in response. I was still pondering on my whole purdey haircut memory. My sister and I would hear the click of the under stair cupboard door open. We would hear the dragging of the dining room chair across the floor tiles in the kitchen and then, we would, in anticipation, stand waiting for the call. On arrival down stairs from the safety of our bedrooms we would see my mother. Her tool of choice in hand....the tongs. We would take it in turns to go first in the hope that she may have improved from our last session the day before. The cries of "mum you are tonging my ear" would be lost in the midst of a Barry Manilow track. It was so much worse than being naughty. It was the price you paid for fashion.

Intriguing isn't it that trends will make up the memories of your youth. Like the afro perm that would happen to my head every three months. I preferred to call it my crash helmet hair. Again it was through my mum's influence that I was introduced. And then of course the memory of spending my early years donning a pair of swimming trunks. My mum had wanted a boy called Mathew....instead she got me. I smiled to myself in the comfort of adulthood.

"Well I began to sample some of my parent's home brew, and then some more, and well then I became both practiced and highly skilled in the art of drunk."

My visit to childhood hairdo's was interrupted. Oh gosh she was still there! Hadn't she finished her little chat with me yet. I'd done the dutiful thing and listened to the person with no friends of her own. She hadn't grabbed my interest, I could tell that not only by my Elvis look but by the fact I was questioning whether her phrasing was grammatically correct. A somewhat alien concept in my every day life. But so obviously oblivious to my disinterest she kept on.

So lardy bloater drunk girl was telling her story and I was trying so hard to not listen.

"Drunk driving....that's what my ban was for. I'd been partying hard with friends, driven home some 30 miles, got to my bedsit and then got back in my car. I drove for ages wanting to get caught really but when the police car clocked me I sped off feeling a bit Cagney and Lacey"

I took a moment as the story continued. Mary Beth Lacey, my idol of the eighties. Her and Christine Cagney, at the park whilst on my tomahawk bike I was them, always doing a slightly clumsy Olga Corbet forward roll in my olive corduroy jeans. They rocked! Anyways I retrained my snarl towards chunky.

"and they caught me"....oops I'd missed a bit. Not a problem she seemed oblivious to that.
"And then what happened?" I asked. (Shit , she had drawn me in I had crossed the line and now was she going to consider me to be fully embraced in the story).

"Well they asked me to get out of the car and I did so with my bra hooked unusually on my belt, kinda of key ring style." (It wasn't a relevant feature of the tale but I quite liked the image the detail encouraged)."And that's why I went to court......"

Chapter Two

I'd managed to sit through the friendly stranger meeting unscathed and I looked up to acknowledge her goodbye but instead the conversation continued, a somewhat depressing prospect. It was weird she seemed thinner and less bubbly. My goodness, had I been sitting there long enough for her to lose weight? She was gesturing towards her mouth. I thought maybe this was instead of a goodbye so I did the same back (now can you see how I may wave at people I don't know during my car journeys.....almost contagious and here I was doing it again.) She did it some more and I returned the now faster movement.

"You have something on your lip" she spoke.

How kind of her to attempt 'embarrassment reduction' for me. It wasn't just something on my lip. I had got latte lipstick!!! The milk moustache, much more common in my youth, it was of course incredibly foamy and arched with perfection. She smiled, I wiped, and she smiled again. Now I felt I owed her...at least to sit for a while longer plus I really was frightened of attempting my window bar stool descent.

"Its not like you see on the films" the conversation had begun again with a random intro. "What's not?" I enquired.

Don't forget I was committed to a minimal chat due to my conscience from the whole latte lipstick rescue. I had a horrible feeling that the part I had missed from the previous conversation was the part I needed to understand this intro. "Its not like you see on the films, detox isn't all hugging and lovely. Its cold and dark and ...."

I butted in...."Detox?" – you see I had missed a good bit!

She replied with an edge of frustration "Yes like I said, that was part of the court's conditions. A year driving ban and to complete a detox program. Only the problem was I was still classed as a minor and from the start it was a 'make it up as you go along' type experience".

She had suddenly grabbed my attention. Dextox units were something I had always been very interested in. I had my own set of theories on the process that should be followed and the philosophy of care that should be offered. I'd spoken often with my friend Jed about the potential to set up a programme. He already had a number of units, you know, care home type stuff. He had always offered me his financial backing if and when the time was right. I felt able to shout up and listen and give the not quite so chunky comedy girl centre stage. I encouraged the story to unfold.....with questions of where and how, the whats and the whys....?

She spoke, "There was no detox unit that was the first barrier. A couple existed in different parts of the country but no where that catered for people under 18. So you see the vision that had been projected to me through do gooders and films I'd seen was far from what I was led in to. I was hammered when I arrived at the 'do gooders' agency that had been assigned the duty of facilitating my path to a clean and straight life. Yes it was in the morning but a party should never end until you're unconscious and so it had been one long ride on the Carlsberg carpet. I was herded through paper work and on to see a 'doctor'. They had so dressed that up! Never would have gone if I knew the doctor was a shrink. What has my leisure activities got to do with mental health.... Even though I was trolleyed I was aware that the 'doctor' office was at the local psychiatric hospital. Feared by many in the town not least for its resemblance to something from the Addams family film set or a Hammer House production. It was a long winding driveway to a collection of dark and scary buildings. I'd been there before twice. Once to a fete where some of the people who lived there were out and about. There was kids as well all packed in a solitary building. I remember it well 'cos I spent the whole afternoon glued to my mum's hip bone and wondering where the little boys legs were hiding that sat motionless in a wheel chair with a make shift banner flapping about in the wind.

The other time I can recall being forced through the Iron Gate way was, to add insult to injury, for a Brownie carol concert. Visiting the individual wards singing a collection of carols in an incredibly out of tune fashion. I (at the time) was not a brownie but had been dragged along with my mum (she wasn't a brownie either!) and my sister (that'll be the one with the brown slightly tired dress, leather belt with old fashioned purse and brown bobble hat) oh how I wished I too was donning that uniform. So the brownies...and me, (I insisted on singing, with no concept of the correct words) begun our choral entertainment. Ward by ward... suddenly I looked around and it appeared I was doing a solo. In fact so solo the rest of the group, including parents, had left the ward to go further into their route. I looked around with desperation scanning the room with a feeling that I may wee my pants through fear. All I could see was old men (at least 100 of them counted through innocent eyes) all with a uniform amount of nose jagglinglys and dirty mouth corners. Trousers – some done up, others not and left so open to the elements. I could see no real people at all. The walls of elderly gentlemen were closing in on me and the invisible protective shield all kids think they have seemed to be turned off. Suddenly I felt hands lifting my bay city rollers sole belt that held up my ill fitting jeans and I was wedgyed out of there by my harassed mum.

So memories of the loony hospital were not fond and there I was about to enter. I was haloed in confusion why I'd be directed to this point but still with the artificial calmness that bourbon tended to install I continued. The shrink was so stereotypical of the mad professor image that immediately gate crashes everybody's mind when anything mental is mentioned. To this day I will never understand why he felt the need to make me strip to my underwear and then proceed to pick out the label of my bra and check it. As I mature my want to understand this action gets far less. The statement of 'mad professor was a dirty pervert' becomes more comfortable in my thoughts. The questions were tedious and repeated. Now I realise the quota I professed to consume daily of alcohol may have encouraged the repetition. In some way hoping that I was making an error in my guesstimation of amounts I drank. But then I just kept repeating the same answers blissfully unaware that the double figures quota in pints matched with the same amount of spirit chasers was actually a large quantity for an evening session. I just knew that was what it was, never entered my head to lie or tone it up or down. Same philosophy has kept me company till now…..truth always the simpler option.

Suddenly I'm moved on from the office and directed through double doors and then some. I arrive in this area full of people milling around and I am ushered into an office type chair in this wide corridor with rooms off it. Later I was introduced to this area as 'the ward'. So I sit there all 12 ish stone of me still kind of riding my

Carlsberg carpet but with slightly less passion and I'm approached by a really smiley lady who introduces herself as Gwen and shakes my hand. She explains that this is a 'ward' and that people are here for lots of different reasons. She continues to ask about my admission and the problems (only ever were problems to others, to me drinking was a talent and a skill that I rocked at). Gwen said that she would do the admission as quickly as possible and that I shouldn't be scared although there were some people who were very poorly and may say unusual things to me. She said she needed to go and fetch a couple of bits and that I should stay sat down. So I did....thinking how friendly and kind she was....just like in the movies!

When I looked up Gwen was approaching me, on her way back at speed. I was surprised at her athletic approach to admissions and smiled as she came nearer. She really was coming at me fast and picking up the pace with every step, I'd like almost to say it was a gallop.....and then she waved something at me. A pen? Wasn't sure but waved right on back. It wasn't a pen and I was able to see that far too clearly as Gwen came flying toward me brandishing a dinner fork. She promptly tried to stab me with it. There was lots of noise. I had such surprised eyes it looked like I had done something majorly wrong whilst plucking my eye brows. I tried to protect myself as I was guessing this wasn't a normal part of the admission process. Then people came running and Gwen was taken away only visible to me through a small window in a room that appeared to have loads of locks on. Gwen wasn't a nurse......Gwen was one of those scary birds who was very poorly....one of many I came across during my stay.

Some bits of that very first day I can remember.....some bits I chose to forget and the rest of the timeless journey has been lost in a rather large amount of detox medication."

Comedy girl was suddenly quiet, maybe even pensive in a kind of William Wordsworth way. I wanted a little more really. I'd got myself comfy. The dismount from the window throne in the coffee shop was far from pending and I was hooked. I asked her to continue... "Hey I'm really interested, what do you remember, it must have been quite a ride?"

One, two, three and she was back in the room. That will be me feeling a tad like Paul McKenna! My face waited, willing a response. I no longer felt a debt to listen from the whole latte lipstick incident and I think she realised her audience was genuine and so comedy girl begun again....

"Ok so here I was 17 years old with already so many lines on my immature face. Each one told a story. I was in charge of myself answered to no one. I'd lived alone pretty much from 16 well officially that was my 16th birthday present all wrapped up in one bag which was my life. But by then I was already settled in. So now, of course I understand that 15 years old is just that little bit to young to know and understand what the world has waiting. But then I was ready and I knew it all. Well I knew it all until that day in March.

So what I remember is being asked the same questions on the ward as I had been all day. I gave the same answers as I had done in the mad professor's office. Then I was handed a rather large gift from the cocktail bar.

"The cocktail bar?" I queried as she paused again for thought.

"Yes the cocktail bar. It was the drug trolley to those who knew better but to me it was the start of something a little bit crazy. I was in a hospital…. allegedly. A nurse (this time I checked) handed me some pills and said take them. So I did. I had no idea what they were. Why I was having them or that the kind of retro shaky dance thing I was doing wasn't just a reaction to being there. It never crossed my mind to ask or to refuse. I'd been brought up with good manners and respect sitting either side of me my whole life and I'd learnt very quickly that to forget them brought difficulty in sitting down for a week. There seemed to be a lot of pills for little me to swallow but I did. What's funny is I can remember them all. The colour and size and shit I can remember the next bit too well.

10…15…maybe even 20 minutes after I'd downed my dose my nose started missbehaving….badly. It was like when I misjudged my forward or backward rolls in a swimming pool. You know when the water goes up your nose and for a minute it hurts."

I nodded….I did know what she meant and I fully understood why all the synchronised swimming team in the Olympics had those ugly nose peg things going on,

She continued "Well like that but so much worse and for so much longer. And with no one to ask or even think about mentioning to. Well no one but 'pretend nurse' Gwen who had now come out of the room with a hundred locks on. She was a prowling around me all the time staring with her eyebrows resting on the top of her eyes. Not my favourite scenery with my foreword roll nose thing going on and then suddenly every thing seemed ok, well actually fantastic really. I wasn't worried about my nose thing in fact I kinda liked it. I wasn't worried about my new home for the night. I just wasn't worried about anything. I was chillin' big time.

It felt like sitting in my favourite chair in my favourite pub (my list of favourite pubs was long and alphabetical) It didn't feel like long before I was handed some more stuff to swallow. I can remember those as well. I also got an explanation. 'You're experiencing a large amount of withdrawal effects and this will help'. I didn't know what they meant.....I do now. So I took the stuff and the rest of that day is gone. That was until I met the drama teacher, another patient staying at the hospital hotel. Interesting first meet and to this day I can't understand quite how we managed to be alone for quite so long....

"What do you mean?" I queried as I didn't want to miss a beat of this story. It was interesting and funny and a little bit scary. A bit like when you see a friend with a new hair do that doesn't tick the pretty box but you're drawn to keep starring at the comedy classic.

She continued.... " Well the one thing I'd noticed from when I first arrived at the 'bedlam wanna be' ward was that I was being watched. Not in a paranoid 'they can see me' way or in a 'crazy lust' way. Just in a 'follow me around' type way. Get me?" She questioned.

I nodded as I think she was describing the level of observation she had been put on by the nursing and medical team. Really close like nearly touching, close but not sit on your lap close and then varying intermittent types like now you see me now you don't or in my experience now I see them...shit now they have run away. Anyhow I digress....I knew what she meant.

"The only time they didn't watch me was the whole nurse Gwen thing and when I became aquainted with the drama teacher. After that there were lots of other times but I never got to know why. "

I clarified my understanding with story girl. I was aware as a nurse that sometimes some people don't quite follow the rules to the book. They follow them more to the point of inconvenience and then suddenly make up new rules to suit. It works most of the time, how it does I'm not to sure but it only takes one brick of the Jenga tower of made up rules to fall. When it does the whole thing comes tumbling down on top of the patient it is built around.

I perched waiting for her to continue and she didn't disappoint with the story that followed.

"So"...she begun," I'm floating my day away and its getting ready for bedtime. Well that's how I saw it. I had a room with two beds in right next to where the nurses all seem to collect for most of the time. I got my wash stuff and floated down to the bathroom area which was communal. Wasn't any different to what I knew as I had spent a long time living in a hostel which was share bedrooms, bathrooms, joints, share everything and I could really tell you a story or to about the lessons I learnt in life there which were far to much fun and a tad early for my innocent eyes......but that's another topic completely.

So I'm washing in front of the sink bit and all lathered up I feel something on my panted arse. Can't see anything for the soap screen I'd covered my face in but I could definitely feel something going on. Instantly I thought how fantastic I'd been given something with a little extra hallucinating kick to it and as a double plus I hadn't paid in money or in kind for the tablet magic. It felt really real which was kinda crazy. So I'm standing there getting a bit busy with my soap suds removal procedure, curiosity testing my patience, and I open my eyes, which were stinging due to the soap overload. Not unlike the whole nostril experience from earlier.

Behind me glaring through the mirror, was a tall dark slightly scary figure female just about with black grey hair and empty stare. I wasn't up for a bad trip as the memories of my last 'not so fabulous' ride through LSD land were still wickedly available. I blinked loads for both the cleansing my stinging eyes reason and for the blink and you change into a best friend rabbit behind me idea. Nothing changed. That was until the figure spoke. Worryingly this was accompanied by much more arse touching.   The voice was monotone and without emotion. "You can catch crabs from the toilet seat in here." Ok I thought kind of random and not your usual hello intro. It seemed like forever but I'm sure it wasn't. Both the realisations came at once, that this was not some poor excuse for a drug induced trip, and the arse thing was not gorgeous, but so obviously connected with scary tall bird. My return to the crab statement was neat and to the point. "Well lady I have some large lobster pincher thing going seriously wrong on my arse at the moment and I ain't taken a piss yet so I suggest you move right away in case it turns round and smacks you full in the face......!" Story teller girl pauses "ah" she said "the confidence that a little something drug like gives you.....you never really can match it in the real world."

I agreed with her sipping my empty latte glass in a swift but convincing manner. I wanted to offer a similar tale to the conversation which had a comedy edge to it. I had been staying with friends not far from the M4, working my way down to Devon, and we were in a night club full of high heel hot pant girls and boys of the gel generation. I had gone off to use the loos which had an entry door with no handle and a hidden step. I'd approached the door, hands positioned for the double push through manoeuvre. As I reached the pushing point of no return the door opened. I tripped over the step, my hands lying to rest on the breasts of the girl who had opened the door to vacate. Not great I thought still trying to control the repercussions of my hidden step-tripping thing. She stared, a little surprised I feel. I gathered composure and balance looked her straight in the eyes, hands still firmly on her boobs and executed the line "Hi, I'm sorry I would usually shake hands." And then continued my journey into the loo..... The moment for that injection of probably not so funny humour was gone. Story teller continued....

"So that was my introduction to the drama teacher. And from then on I was to find myself in the unwanted position of 'her bitch' or so she convinced herself and with that came all sorts of trouble.... for me. I didn't know what the phases being banded about meant in relation to the drama teacher and me. Obsession, compulsion, psychotic thoughts, morbid jealousy and delusions. I wasn't sure if they were invitations to join a small tester session for weird and wonderfully named 'tabs and trips'. I'll have some of that I thought in a good ole' fashioned try anything once approach. I have, in my maturity, grown more accustomed to the terms. All I knew was that when she was around she was sure to try and cop a feel, stalk me, want me and in some ways haunt my every move. The arse thing, that just got more wrong. Sometimes it made the nurses watch me and sometimes they forgot. That wasn't my favourite but as I grew stronger and angrier it seemed less of a issue. In fact towards the end of my stay it became more of a sport.

So for the next few days I can remember some things but not all. I can remember being visited by the friend. I had pinned her up against the wall the night before I arrived at Hammer Horror House hospital. She had thought it was a good idea to pour my half full (always the optimist) bottle of beer down the sink. I, on the other hand, had disagreed. The Jekyll in me that used to arrive unannounced when I'd had a skinfull, launched a sewer mouth attack in her direction. This was whilst she was cemented to the wall by my clutch. Ugly...even to think about it now. Ashamed of course and never enough sorrys will make it prettier. So I carry that along with a number of outtakes which maybe keeps me clean....for now.

Anyway she was visiting, my first full day and I was sitting at a table. I was shaking...big time. I watched stuff dance in front of me. I picked up pieces of paper and stones only visible to me. Some moved, some didn't. It was an ok feel, just different. I didn't feel scared. I didn't really feel at all. She sat down and we began to talk.... I think. Or maybe only in my head and the voice to her was a stranger. I was handed some more pills, they came frequently and varied in colour. So like the sucker to the system I was, I swallowed. And we carried on. I felt something weird going on, dizzy ...? Well a bit I suppose. More numb really then I found myself being carried and a bit dragged into the room opposite where I sat only a few minutes before. I could here everything, couldn't see a lot but I could hear my friend. She was, as anyone would be, a tadge confused. Lots of poking started happening, I could tell it wasn't the drama teacher, her favoured areas were left well alone. It was my eye lids and my ears and my chest. A bit of face slapping too and still unsure of the value in that but hey good for them.

I heard someone address my friend. " It's ok....." I laid there thinking well it's kind of not that ok. They told her I could hear but that I had reacted to the medication and that I would be alright in a while. I was screaming out how long is a while? But of course no one could hear me. My lips, my eyes my hands, nothing moved. I wanted to say to my friend to go. My body was paralysed but my mind so wasn't. It did wear off ...eventually but I never got to understand why or how that had occurred. No one told me and of course then I didn't know there was room to ask. I thought maybe it was all part of what should happen. Thinking about it now I am so pleased I didn't get a run down of the 'what's going to happen next' list."

"Would you have stayed?" I butted in, not meaning to but I almost felt I was living the whole thing with comedy girl.

She answered..."No...but I didn't know I could leave, and I'm not sure I could as I found out later.... The hard way."

Chapter Three

We seemed to come to a natural pause and so I took the opportunity to invite story teller to have another drink. I did a hair flick in the direction of the waitress and then a more assertive wave, come here move. I had to. The dismount from the window throne was not an option and she looked sort of helpful....that or a bit stoned. I asked if she wouldn't mind getting us some drinks and she obliged. "I'll have another latte please and a mocha choca loca coca (oh god I couldn't stop) styli type drink." There was really nothing cosmopolitan or continental in that failed attempt with far too many addons. She smiled and returned with two filter coffees. Not going to argue that minor oversight. We sipped and then the story continued.

"My friend came back you know. Once a week, every week, for the whole stay. That was like a solid thing that I knew was ok and reliable. Had a couple of other mates come. They'd helped me build a foundation of growing up memories that, as adults we recall with such pride. It was the era of house parties and a comedy gift in the form of 'girls on top'. It was where middle of the road was not an option and the more outrageous you could be the more excepted it was. One had a proper grown up job that we didn't really understand and.... Still don't. The other done singing like instead of working which was majorly cool and a bit celeb. She knew people who lived on my poster wall that I kissed. Most importantly though these were my friends, not just for the good times.

Someone else from where I was working came to try and see me. I say try because I was having none of it. Just before my admission....yuk I hate the sound of it. I had been seeing quite a bit of one of the nurses at work;

I was a carer for people, you know in wheelchairs and stuff. I did loads of nights which worked well cos' I used to bring in a large amount of tinnies and then piss the night away. That was until one night I was, I reckon half way through my third run of the 'dirty dancing' video with the curious but sexy 'no body puts baby in the corner' Patrick Swaze line. That's all I remember until I was woken by noise and a presence in the lounge room where I had made a little sleeping area.

My eyes opened to find my manager and two other workers dodging beer cans to get a better view of me. I had also placed piles of wet washing all over the floor as a way of keeping me busy through the night so as not to fall asleep. Guessing that wasn't my best plan ever. The manager who was not on shift had been called to come from the town where she lived as no one could get in the building (security conscious me!) I'd fallen asleep and it was now about 7.30 or 8am. I immediately realised this was not going to be the best bit of my CV in future, collected my beer cans and left. Anyway the point is I had been hanging around with one of the workers who seemed quite friendly but a bit unusual. She kept asking me to stay the night and I wasn't thinking that was my favourite. She was a bit too motherly for my liking. Now I'm guessing she thought maybe we could have a kind of thing going on but then it just felt weird and I'd totally missed any come on she was offering.

Actually it was proper weird. In fact I'll tell you what it was like. It was the same feel as I had had when I was 15 at school. A caretaker was chasing me down the corridor with a cinzano bottle in his rubber-gloved hand. Yes it was mine, well mine and a girl in the year below and yes we had stored it in the high up cystern at the end toilet in the old block of the school. And yes ok it had flooded the whole toilet block and outside corridor but it wasn't intentional. This girl and me had been having a little drink prior to registration. She was a beautiful looking girl and after she left school her life was really waiting for her. She had a job on T.V. It's sad to think about her now though. When she died I read it in the paper. She committed suicide. There are some crazy changing lanes of destiny.

But that isn't why I had the weird feel. That came when I ran, still trying to escape rubber glove cinzano man, straight into the arms and overly exaggerated childbearing hips of the PE teacher. One of three and with each I had a not so friendly relationship. She kind of marched me towards her office door; she was head of year, which year I have no idea. I'd only once been this close to her before. It was when she was demonstrating how I should throw the discus. I was caccooned in her grasp whilst she rotated my hips to and fro. It wasn't gorgeous and intriguing as I had been throwing discus for a couple of years reaching a national level. She on the other hand had not, but still her hands were glued to me in an awkward embrace of no gain. So this was the second contact with hips aplenty. She took me into her room and shut the door.... K chink like a comic strip lock. She instructed me to sit on the low down comfy chair with no arms. I mean the chair had no arms I didn't have to amputate mine or anything.

The chair was next to her office window looking into a garden courtyard where no one went. She started to talk to me in a soft gentle tone I was not accustomed to. I was waiting for the telling off about the whole flooding thing and it just didn't come. It seemed she tried to get me to talk to her, to open up a little but I had nothing to tell. Yes, like I said it was difficult and yes school was a good place to be but it wasn't a story and anyway other teachers had been asking questions so I'd done that answering thing once already, well sort of.

So the hips got up from behind her desk and made their way over to the other comfy seat which was touching mine. She sat them down and continued her conversation, which was all too one sided. I sat and stared at the tired flowers in the courtyard. In one swift kendo type movement I was pulled to the side and my head found its self side-saddle on her lap. She started stroking my hair and my face was being buried in her lady garden in a wrong way. My first thought was that I guessed this wasn't going to be where she hid her sweets, quickly followed by an exit manoeuvre. I was out of that office and down the corridor before she realised I was no longer her lap cat. That was how come I had the weird creepy bit over friendly but wrong feel. She never discussed it or spoke with me again which I was very happy with…unusual though I thought.

So I had the same feel with the worker lady who was a bit too motherly friendly. So when she came to see me I ran down the corridor (I am hoping aided by the copious amounts of medication) shouting "I can't see her she has hairy legs". Fortunately this drew enough attention to act as a deterrent for her visits but because of the general madness on the ward it did little more than that. I did not pick up any extra meds for some hypothetical illness an over keen shrink may think I had. I had another visitor too, she came with a towel and a bar of soap."
"Who was she?" I engaged…

"She was a teacher from school, she was the grown up that I felt I owed the world to. Now I know I owed her for her silence which cost me a harsh lesson in trust but again that's for another time. I liked the soap she bought me, it was pearl, it smelt nice. I liked the towel too. It was dusky pink and it was waffled. They were mine to keep, that and a couple of pairs of shorts and tops made up my wardrobe. So anyway she used to come once a week as well."

Chunky had referred to the teachers a couple of times now. It was like she opened the floor for questions but before I could ask them she stole the moment away. I tried to gain more clarity, for the story? Not really I suppose, more for a sense of what comedy girl was about. "This teacher, the helpful one, she sounds interesting?"

An air of tension smothered comedy girl's face. "She didn't help me, well I thought she did, but she didn't."

Ok so I had been dealt a riddle. I wasn't sure what she meant by her double negative statement thingy. "What do you mean?"

"Look" she replied, agitated by the interruption. "You think when you're little that grown ups sort stuff out. That they are the ones to keep you safe. There should never be any pleasure gained through a child's fear, never any glory or false admiration. My friends knew something about it was wrong but we were kids. I have the same friends now. Today her name is not said with warmth from their adult lips.

You see She asked me a couple of times what was going on. I suppose I hinted at the truth although it was often clouded in the belief that I was at fault. I was in trouble but not on purpose. Maybe if I tried harder if I wanted to I could talk nice, write nice, you know, stuff like that. That was how it was depicted to me. The rest she didn't need a commentary for. It was usually mapped out on my face from the night before.

Like I said, it wasn't her secret to keep. I was also into martial arts so perhaps for those who never asked there was an avenue of explanation. You know like a heavy training session or something I suppose. Despite my pleas sometimes the teacher bird would phone my parents. It was a long time ago. As with everyone then, people believed discipline was the key. That always resulted in a difficult time. I'd been thrown out of all my other classes and so really the only contact I had was with her. She had said to the headmaster that she would watch over me because I was no longer able to attend any classes. That'll be the naughty side of me. It was cool I suppose. I got to do work all day with no one bothering me or poking their nose in. Most of the time I doodled or did maths stuff. That was easy, it made sense. Actually when I say naughty I may be toning it down slightly. I may have been a handful. Full up of cheekiness but, never nastiness. Lots of laughing, the joker in the pack of teenager playing cards.

She'd kept me back from class one day, the teacher. She said it was to discuss how my speech was. She reckoned it had gone down hill. I didn't know what she meant at all, I told her I wasn't doing the public speaking competition that was held in the library. It was that time of year. I didn't like stuff like that. I found it hard and I'd had enough of that stuff in class anyway. Id had months of being made to read out loud in front of the other kids. It was like a daily matinee performance from the odd one. Teacher bird didn't mean the competition anyway. She was proper talking about me and I didn't understand. She reckoned all the teachers had noticed and they'd all had a chat about it. Me and my friends hadn't noticed....but that's because kids don't make the world complicated. They leave that job to the grown ups. The teacher bird said it was difficult to understand me sometimes. She said it had deteriorated. I didn't know what that meant. Didn't care much either. The bit that wasn't gorgeous was that she finished up the conversation with the 'I've phoned your parents' line. My heart sank. Sometimes It felt like she was sowing seeds and then watching them grow. She knew the score, I know she did.

She kept me back late at school then dropped me off home. I asked her a hundred times not to but she said she had to, that it was her job. I said I would be fine to walk. I didn't want her to leave me there as she had done so many times before. I liked her a lot. She spoke to me nice.

You see when I walked in that night they were waiting. I knew they would be. Their school of thought being that this, once again, was my fault or my doing. That if it was made to hurt enough I would stop and I would be mended. Phrase after phrase I repeated encouraged by the belief that I was wrong. I couldn't make my words clearer. I was making them worse with each strike...and then I stopped. I wasn't mended. I didn't talk much after that not at home or at school because it hurt.

The next day she called me into her room from my desk position outside her class. This was my everyday seat. She was marking work and so did not look up. She asked me why I had left my desk during lesson time. She had obviously clocked me moving around outside her room where she was teaching first years. I explained I had gone to get some tissue. My nose had done some bleeding. She looked up from her marking. It had far too much red pen tracing the scribbled work in front of her. My eye was black, my nose was broken and still a drop or two of blood escaping, my face told the rest of the story. "Ok?" she said "Was that last night, keep some tissue with you" It was a statement not a question. I liked her. I thought she was making it all ok. That it was all ok, that things were meant to be like that because she never said they weren't. I now know she wasn't doing anything but some times she said kind stuff. Anyway that's the story. Don't ask me again it's forever ago."

Comedy girl was keen to get on with the show. She had answered my questions. I regretted asking them now. I didn't need to know that stuff. I needed to shut up and listen a bit.

"What followed were days and nights of busy head busy legs and very little sleep. When I did sleep they woke me up as I was often half way off the bed. Not a problem to me but to them it wasn't the tidy look they seemed to be after. I would often fall out of bed too and stay asleep. Again this was not unusual as at home I would always wake up on the floor but through my stay it seemed to be a point of unwanted interest in my rehabilitation so they called it. The first few days I had a nurse watching me bath it made me cry. I don't know why but I felt so silly and so naked! Sometimes I see her now, she was a student then, she is a ward sister now in the general hospital. Sometimes I want to say hello to her and tell her she was nice to me when the world felt wrong. I never do tell her, in fact I have never spoke to her. My eyes just fall to the floor and I walk by.

One day I came to tell the nurses that I didn't feel very well…. maybe the eighth or ninth day I can't remember. I know I had been promoted to the dormitory and I didn't get followed hardly at all. I never really said much about whether I felt ok or not and so it seemed that if I did say something they would believe me...and why not...I learnt quickly the same didn't apply to everyone. So I came towards the nurses' collection point area and I got a bit more hurried. It seemed miles away down the ward corridor and getting further out of my sight. I was carrying a can of coke. I reached to put it on the table near to me as I remember thinking I don't want to make a mess. Unfortunately the only thing that met the table was me moving face down to the floor. So much for my tidy try! Don't know how long I was on the floor but I knew I had blood pressure things being velcroed on and I was placed in a position like a live sculpture. There was a lady I didn't know who spoke sort of broken English, she was ordering the nurse to do something nurse like and the nurse who I had seen before was telling her no not until the fit had stopped. Oh how exciting until I realised they were talking about me! When I was allowed to get up I asked for some paper towel to clear my coke mess up. There was a screen around my landing point. How long does it take to get a screen? I didn't want to know. I was guessing longer than a second or two which was how long I hoped the whole show had lasted. I didn't talk to anybody about what happened and I didn't want to. I went and stayed on my bed."

Comedy girl had said nothing funny for ages. I was still drawn into the whole narrative episode but it seemed that the stuff she felt sad about when it happened she told me in a sad way, the stuff that made her smile she told me with humour and the stuff that made her cross she expressed in the emphasised dialogue of swearing. I enquired if she felt ok

"Yes" she said ".... there was funny stuff too" (had she heard my thoughts again? like the original 'don't sit near me' statement which was made available to her when she removed her Bart Simpson ear muffs?)

She continued. "There is some funny stuff that happened....as I got sober and clean I got naughty. And actually even before the very steep sliding scale of medication reduction and end of the injection program......now that was something worth a mention. Every day it seemed I had injections in my upper outer quadrant.... I say it like I know what it meant. To me it was top of arse cheek either side on alternate days. They hurt and drama teacher always seemed to get a ring side seat....guessing it was the arse thing but never curious to have that confirmed. One day something went a bit wrong with the injection. I know that because there was lots of 'are you OKs?' and running and whispering. Didn't bother me any and it hurt just like any other day. My knee did something a bit weird when I walked. Couldn't help it doing it and actually it lasted for ages but I never thought there may be a connection. Funny really 'cos even now if I'm tired or I have a cold and stuff in it comes and goes when I walk. Some things are better left unexplored. I put it down to coincidence. Every day they would offer me pain relief for it and I had physio loads. I continued to refuse the pain stuff 'cos I couldn't find any other way to help them understand it didn't hurt, not proper, not enough to have medicine. My mum had brought me up with the philosophy of no fuss....ever. if your leg falls off on the way to school pick it up and pop it in your rucsac and make sure you're not late type teaching which really I have carried on and plus it really wasn't a problem.... to me. Everyone makes mistakes don't they? The innocence that trust encourages is sometimes scary to consider but for me it was how it was.

I spent days trying to bribe anyone who would listen to bring me in liqueurs, somehow I thought they would magically stop my cravings and additional tense feel that I had as my companion. I offered my telly and my personal stereo that was all I had to offer but to me it was a fair swap. I saw the word alcohol on some wipe things in the medical looking room, so, on a mission I would try and sometimes succeed in getting my hands on them. They didn't taste good at all and that little stunt cost me a good hard shove against the wall, out of telling eyes way, and a fist in my face, from one of the more slightly old school nurses. She was hard but hand on heart I listened but then it was a style I was not alien to.

I met a fella called Dog. He seemed to have some big time drink issues but it was weird 'cos he was allowed to go to the pub all day and come back at nights steaming. I think he was there to protect him for a court date but when I say that now it sounds like I got sucked in to a big fat fib. Didn't mind too much thought 'cos I would wait for him to return off his trolley and then in my youthful approach would ask if he fancied some cards. Late at night it always feels ok for the stakes to be high. Add that to his inability to function cos of the alcohol intake and I was on to a sure thing. I enjoyed cards anyway....it kept me out of trouble prior to my entry to ....detox. Well it kept me in pocket, as did my pool playing. Some people would suggest I was taking advantage financially of a drunk in-patient...I call it resourceful!

As the drugs became less so the discomfort became more. My mind was sober and open to thought. A whole new concept I hadn't experienced without artificial comfort for a long time. I didn't feel very with it. I sat alone a lot or with some of the helper people who seemed to think it was really cool that I would play the games with them for hours on end and chat about regular stuff. Never talking about proper more about the telly or what ever they fancied really. When I sat in the lounge type room I would look at this clay model. Horrible ugly little thing perched on the side. It looked a bit like a skeleton face if you squinted. One day I asked what it was. And one of the friendly helper people told me a patient had made it. She was a young girl with anorexia, I only knew that it meant thin people thought they were chunky. When she was staying on that ward she had made it with an art person. It was her answer to the request they had made for her to make her image of pretty and perfect. I looked a little more at the figure silently guessing that she wasn't quite cured at the point of her artistic challenge....some messed up chick she must have been! I kept my opinion to myself almost but a little bit fell out of my mouth.

That was one thing I had noticed during my stay. People staying there could get away with saying anything there. Lots of it I found really funny...weird but funny."

I stared at comedy girl in a telling way.... These people were ill, they were disturbed, the things they said were probably part of their symptoms....

She replied "yeah and I was 17 jammed in a loony bin; the stuff I heard was fuckin' funny. Anyway I was disturbed....ok not by illness, more by the ever increasing unwanted attention by scary drama teacher lady who by this stage kept standing in front of me doing a dance. You know the one you see old rocker girls do at pub gigs which is never going to be sexy not even through drunken disoriented eyes. Always looks like a pension person porn production but with clothes on.

Sets my gag reflex off every time. Not sure what the purpose of the whole silent dance serenade thing was but jeez she kept it up.

Hey, there was a woman, I can remember this so well. She had OCD that was all I knew. Didn't know what it was but it made her hands red raw all the time. So much so she had to keep washing them.....like loads. And then cleaning down taps, tables, you name it. I found it really cool that I would leave stuff in a mess and turn around and like a cleaning fairy she was there tidying as I went. Now I realise that's why I was like her worst favourite person. Then I thought she just didn't like me which made things interesting. Some times her hands would bleed. Yes I know.....they bled because she washed them too much but then I thought it was the other way round. That was until the day I realised! Same day as I was given a task as part of her rehabilitation. I felt ever so important. She had been working with some helper who used to arrive every so many days to help her leave her washing in the machine and not watch it. They had progressed to the stage where she had to ask someone (that'll be me) to put it in the dryer for her whilst she went out.

I'm under no illusion of just how difficult that must have been for her but then I just didn't get it at all and because she was always really nasty to me I though I'd do pay back. So off she goes having checked the washing machine door about 10 times and I'm left in charge. As I mentioned the penny had dropped that day that she had a big cleaning thing going on and found it big time hard. So when the machine stopped I was waiting. No-one else watching not even drama teacher. She had been put in the locked up room and I don't think the shouting I heard when it happened were cheers...not sure. So anyway she was out of the picture for a while. Luxury in itself. The timer on the machine clicked off and so my role in rehabilitation of the cleaning nasty woman began! I pulled out every single item which was in that machine and placed it on the floor (that was the bit of the task I added in with no one telling me) I then danced on the top of the lot, making sure each bit of clothing got a bit of my dance all to itsself. Loved it every minute of it. I then placed the whole load in the dryer as I had been asked to do and found my way back to the lounge room.

From that day I never once cared what the OCD woman said to me or how she was 'cos I'd danced on her washing and she didn't know it. Fortunately I never felt the need to tell her what I had done in complete detail; I'm guessing it wouldn't have sped up her recovery."

I sat opened mouthed. Comedy girl was a bitch! She noticed my freeze frame expression and rounded off that story with the fact "yeah and still proud of it!"

"When the sliding scale of medication had been reduced almost to nothing I found my self with a foul mouth and a disgusting attitude towards the world in general. It was about the same time as the results of some blood they had taken came through to do with damage to my liver. I was taken to a room where I think they were trying to discuss the severity of what I had done to my body through having the odd tipple. There was lots of statistics thrown at me of which I had no interest or understanding of. I'd slipped comfortably into the costume of a very stroppy teenager with no respite from my thoughts or nightmares that didn't seem to ration themselves to my sleep. 'You 'll be dead within three years' was a quote I remember to which I said well leave me alone 'cos all you're doing is wasting valuable drinking time. It's scary how practical that statement felt to me at the time. Needless to say I found it hard to engage. I couldn't understand why I was still there at the time; I didn't consider this was only the start of the detox program and behind the scenes people,...not sure who, were trying to find a placement that would take a minor to complete a full rehabilitation program.... glad I didn't know.

Chapter Four

I had these meeting things what were nasty. I seemed to get one with lots of proper professional unapproachables sat in a row sometimes. One of the nurses thought it appropriate to mention that I wore socks and no shoes outside in the meeting thing one day. That wasn't helpful, I didn't like her much. She never spoke to me. She said I refused to wear shoes at all and that maybe this was something a little bit mental like. She used bigger words, but that's what she meant. I sat silently. They discussed it with each other and like Miss 'Invisible' I did tennis court action with my head. It was just like when the spectators move from shot to shot, only I was doing towards each person who spoke. When I came out of the room which I hated going in I went and sat on my bed....doing some of that thinking thing. I wasn't allowed outside much at all, and only with a nurse anyway so I got really excited to walk round the ground to have some air. Funny really as now I always have to be able to escape outside just so I can smell the air sometimes, probably 'cos I'm an outside girl rather that anything to do with that experience but for story purposes we can link it...makes for the drama.

Anyway I sat on my bed and for that minute I felt sad inside. I didn't want to tell anybody I didn't have a pair of shoes to wear. The only ones I had I had made a hole in, probably during one of my comedy trips. I always was falling over, never grew out of it. One evening I was on a bit of a date and I was playing snooker when suddenly my lace hooks on my boots got caught up together both the left and right shoe....yes it was clever but with this came the instant fall flat on my face so to my date for the night at the other end of the snooker table it was a case of now you see her now you don't. Not my best do you fancy me move I've ever executed I can tell you. Anyway the pleasure that comes when you're sidetracked by reminiscing.... So I'm on my bed in the Hammer House Hospital and I'm thinking. I don't have any shoes to wear and I don't want to tell anybody so I had been outside and inside in my socks but not for anything mental. I wasn't allowed to go to the town shops by myself and I couldn't go with a nurse in my socks, I knew that much. Couple that with my pride and that I didn't have any money it was all (like not that much) in my bank account. I was ashamed of me....

Had some extra pills for the 'not wearing shoes' thing. Didn't know that at the time, all I was sure of was that I had lots of pills to take sometimes and one or two on other occasions. When they gave me the medicine I didn't ask why, I just thought it was for the drinking thing. It made me feel funny....not really very nice. Bit dancy really like I couldn't keep still and at night I had a huge nightmare thing going on which wasn't my favourite at all. Woke up so scared I nearly weed in my pants. Had a big look around and the comfort you would normally find when you realised that you were in your own room didn't come. More the thump of 'still in the loony bin'.

After a couple of days had gone past with the new dancy uncomfortable and tired me, one of the nurses approached me with some 'paperwork'. I wasn't interested or sure what it was and what it was for but she insisted that I fill it in....something to do with the hospital and sickpay. Wasn't certain what to do with the forms...a big chunky pile of them tricking you into thinking they were an easy read booklet. So I filed them in the bin which was outside of the ward dormitory. Later that day they arrived in front of me, this time with a table slap and a pen to help in the process. And there I sat, pen in hand, leaning on my beano comic read poised for action. Time stood still in the hospital. It didn't really matter if it was the morning or evening, people were around doing stuff. No idea what the stuff being done was but if ever I did approach somebody to use the phone or unlock a door they were all really busy all of the time. It gave me more reason never to ask 'cos I had all the time in the world. Even at night there was business and noise and sitting in chairs with sheets on having a snore. I don't know how long I was there, for probably something like a week-long hour. I can remember being on the first page about 2 thirds of the way down. I had filled one question in, it had felt like a long time doing it. I didn't like filling in forms, or writing, or reading, really. My only like at school had been when we got to make up a story. Loved those but often they came back with phrases like 'needs to concentrate on grammar'. 'Spelling poor' and 'if she spent as much time in the real world as in her imagination she would do well'. My mum had always said I was never bored, always making things or pretending to be something playing for hours with or without company; still the same now, just a splash of Peter Pan never hurts.

So I'm there with the form, one answer down, 100 odd to go. The same nurse was on her way back like the whole entire form filling police just marching toward me in a 'hope its done and back in the over size envelope' way.

"So all done?" she presumed, hand at the ready to receive the form. It was like a relay race exchange Olympic style with the form as our baton. She threw a glance to the table and saw my proud work. "Really this needs to be done today, it's for your benefit, so why aren't you doing it?"

"I am" I stated, "look...."

She pulled up a chair next to me, felt quite nice really as I had only spoken to a few people when the tablets were being given out. They asked if my mouth was empty and of course the helper people who played games and chatted about telly and bits like that.

"Can you read the form ok?" She asked.

Didn't know what to say to that really. I hated reading and was slow at it. But this form made no sense and I wasn't able to read it well at all. ...but yes I could read the form...just not very well. I wasn't about to volunteer myself for the 'dumma of the year' competion so I opted for the easy answer.... I said nothing at all.

She asked again it if wanted a hand doing the form. "Yes" I said "please." Much better question for me to answer. She was called Abby and she said tomorrow would be good to do the form together. That suited me. I was in one big long day anyway.

Abby found me in the morning quite early and we went off to the table and chair bit where we sat down. There weren't many people around...maybe cos I wasn't looking. I felt comfy with Abby which was kind of weird but ok. She read the form out to me which made things a lot better, but when I tried to write the stuff I couldn't very well remember how to write it. Very quickly Abby decided she would write the form also. I was trying to remember when the last time I wrote something down was. Couldn't, had spent the last two years of school and then some drunk.... all of it which was cool, but not I suppose, in a scary 'I can't remember how to write' way.

Abby was nice to talk to, she was kind to me with the form thing and when she had finished she didn't go straight away, she talked to me. She asked me if I wanted to go outside for a while for a walk and I of course said yes (over excited by the slightest change in a timeless routine). "Go get your shoes on then and I'll wait here."

Abby had been on holiday so had missed the shoe thing a couple of days ago and now Abby 'nice lady' would become one of them when I made no attempt to get shoes.

"Have they told you to come and talk to me about shoe wearing?" I said to her...now feeling silly that I thought she was comfy ok. She looked puzzled. "From that meeting thing I had about not wearing shoes and that being mental and stuff?"

She showed no acknowledgement of those clues I had given her. Abby said she was just going to let the staff know she would be leaving the ward and then come back. 'Yeah right' I thought, but then she tapped me on my shoulder letting me know she was ready.
"Come in your socks if you want to, come on lets get some air". Abby was proper cool.

We walked around the grounds which were big and green. Some of the land was used for other stuff so people in cars would drive by staring at you as you walked, a bit like it was a hobby...."wanna come and stare at the mad people as we drive around?".

We sat on a bench for a bit....that was cool too. Abby said to me "you don't have any shoes to wear do you?" I stayed looking straight ahead "nope" I answered. We didn't have to talk anymore about that, we just sat and smelt the air. I do know that from then on I didn't have to have the mental pills for the shoe thing so in turn I didn't get scared at night to go to sleep for the company that may break in to my dreams. Didn't feel dancey inside either. Abby was cool. I liked her.

Being on the ward became nothing more than habit. I kept myself to myself and I wasn't really sure what, if anything, was the plan from now on. I knew that the nurses had spoken about a detox unit I would be going to. I wasn't involved in the conversations so I just carried on.

Oh I almost forgot....the whole pregnant thing!"

"You were pregnant" I echoed, "what do you mean what happened?"

"No I wasn't pregnant....but at the time I couldn't remember where I had been for the last two or three months prior to getting in the hospital. I knew like that I'd seen mates and bits like that but I didn't know the where's or the when's or anything really. I knew I had eaten a bag of Bovril crisps during that time however they didn't seem even slightly impressed by that. I had favoured a more liquid diet making sure that I always had a pint of milk first and then Guinness for the iron and so on. It's funny really, I was known for my pint of milk as the kick off drink and at the local pub I frequented daily it would be on the bar waiting as I arrived. They were a lovely couple who owned it, they even arranged for me to have an 18th birthday party there with a cake and stuff and the rest of the people who propped up the bar. It was a bit of a tongue in cheek occasion really as they had been serving me for a long while before so they were kind of saying we knew you were under age but you're not now. I didn't have

Gellespi Donks

the heart to tell them it was actually only my 17th birthday....the cake looked to good! That was also the venue for meeting the one who took away my virginal status. That was farce. I knew him from being in the pub and one day he said did I want to go and look at his record collection. I was a big fan of music and readily agreed. I know what you're thinking but then and now I take things a bit literally and of course when I got there I asked where the records were. He just looked at me, and laughed. I think he thought I was taking the piss which of course I wasn't. I didn't like him much; I certainly didn't find him attractive. I stayed a while then he let me leave. Got back to the room I called home at the time and had a nose bleed. I knew from girl chats that after the thing there was blood. It was only later, as in years later that I understood blood ordinarily did not come from your nose.....it makes me smile, the innocence of youth and literal thinking.

But I digress, so no I wasn't pregnant but when I couldn't recall anything about the previous 2 or 3 months and I had no menstrual cycle then I guess alarm bells sounded for the nurses. So I did a pregnancy test. I didn't like doing it and what was crazy funny was out of all the bits that had happened at the loony bin and how I was that was the thing that made me feel cheap. Not for long but it adds emotion to the story don't you think."

I was bemused by comedy girl's dismissive manner. She was very matter-of-fact and without injury visible to the listener. Recounting her experiences with such detail...when she wanted it but as a commentary...intriguing.

She began to speak again, "so next thing that happen was they moved me on to a different ward. I felt that my little bit of world had been smashed. I had learnt to feel

46

comfortable with some of the staff and they had I think learnt a bit about me and then suddenly I was put some where different."

"How come?" I queried.
"Well", she adjusted her seating position and this drew my eye. Where had the chunky lardy elephant butt gone I found myself wondering…which is wrong in every sense but her whole figure had shrunk. I am positive that nobody had run into the coffee house and stolen chunky girl's hips but now this slight figure was in her place. I realised that the whole arse wondering thing had made me miss the start of the explanation as to the ward move.

I stopped her, "sorry I missed that". What a difference from when we first met and I tried every avoidance in the book! The thing was I actually didn't want to miss any bit of her story.

She continued "its ok, I was moved because well I fell out with someone. …actually before I start that bit I've just thought of something that haunts me still about the first ward I was on. It was awful and I sometimes try and replay it in my mind to get a better story ending. It was one thing that really made me feel frightened."

At last my comedy storyteller was with emotion, albeit fear, but still it was emotion. I encouraged her to continue by the sarcasm with which we appeared to mimic each other's injection into the conversation…"what you? Scared?"

She began to explain…

"Yes, it was one day out of the big long day I was in during the 'detox sliding scale = you're not having as much medication as yesterday' saga. I can remember seeing this lady. Kind of almost as if she was in a coma. She did walk around.... not far but her eyes were empty and her hair dishevelled. She was proper posh I think though and even with her somewhat untidy presence her clothes, well, all of her, looked expensive. She didn't really eat or drink. Sometime she had a visit from a man. I think it was her husband as they did that thing that tired married couples do. You know the look at each other thing rather than engage and the niceity conversation that follows when they have nothing left to talk about apart from divorce. Anyway this one day there was so much noise. It was like real life screaming which wasn't coming from any horror film one of the many very disturbed patients insisted on watching.... over and over. The screaming was coming from posh lady's room (she had her own room, not 'cos she had paid private though, I don't think). The screamin' was really scared sort and deep rather than the 'I've seen the man of my dreams' girl scream. And then she came out of the room. She was doing more movement than I had ever seen her do before. She had a nurse helper on each arm and someone holding her head. I'm guessing it wasn't in case her head fell off. She didn't so much walk as she was dragged down the corridor, still desperately screaming and struggling to get away. She was crying too...bit of a double whammy really. I don't think I ever saw someone so upset. Well apart from the fat people at funerals on the telly from other countries who wail ever so loud and then fall to their knees head in hands. She was far sadder than that. I could hear her screaming even after the ward doors had closed and it rang through the hollow corridors for what seemed like minutes.

The nurses were going about their business, well the ones that were left. Loads had gone with posh lady like a convoy filtering out of the door at the end of the long and gloomy corridor. It was an awful feeling. When someone sounds that scared and distressed you want to go to him or her, to help them and make it all alright. I couldn't think why she was like that or where she was going but it didn't seem that she wanted to, I know that much. Sat for ages after she had left the ward just thinking about it and how I did nothing to help her. It was all really confusing 'cos in the hospital you are there to be made better and to feel safe but that screamin' thing which was going on out of her did not depict either was the case...and I had just sat and watched the helpers...helping?"

"So where did she go? Had she had bad news?" I was pacifying the story really as I had a pretty good idea what was coming next.

"Well, I didn't find out 'til much later where she had been for the couple or three hours she was not on the ward. I learned this over time and from the conversations staff had with each other with disregard to any confidentiality that may now be present. She had been for 'treatment'! That's what they called it. Treatment meant electric shocks being forced in to you through comedy horror sponge pads on the end of wired-up sticks. It sound's like torture doesn't it?"

Comedy girl's face was looking back at me, still with the innocent confusion that comes with the belief that hospital and doctors know best and make you better.... and care for you.

She continued "When posh lady returned it seemed even more scary than her departure. The ward doors boomed open both at once and nurses half carried half dragged her frozen legs through the entrance. She seemed asleep but with her eyes glazed open. Empty stare still very present. Her hair still dishevelled but on the sides of her head were marks. Quite distinctive and rounded, the size of the bottom of a small drink bottle I suppose. The marks looked sore really red and screaming. Her feet were the last thing to enter her bedroom and I didn't see her again til late that night. I think she only had one more treatment after that with much the same drama, the screaming how ever was more tired and her struggle was defeated before she begun. As a teenager I knew that the treatment was sucking her spirit away, her last fight for her life. When the treatment stopped I never heard her scream like that or cry or struggle, she seemed too busy getting better. I wonder though if she felt better inside or was just too scared to let anyone see because when she had let them in she was held down, drugged and tortured. Much the same as we read with horrified eyes in our newspapers. "

The experience that story teller depicted had left a dent, you could see it. Almost as if her childhood beliefs and rules that make up the world had been challenged that day as it seemed had many more in her 'cini' film memories of her stay. I wanted her to know I was getting it, the feelings she must have had. I told her about a time I was in a canteen at a work place I had to visit and that as the staff queued for their food in a closed silence that accompanies lines where no one wants to chat . I saw someone I had known years previously. A posh lady in the queue on her own. She looked ok but lines on her face told their own story. She had slight scarring on the side of her head more discolouring really. It took me back to when I had seen her before, she had been climbing a mountain that life had put in her way. As I chased the memory she looked up from her queue space and through my gaze. I looked right back at her and realised what had been stolen had never been replaced."

My new companion and I pause for a sip of cold but still classy coffee. She knew I got the feel, as did I for her. We didn't need to elaborate; you don't when you get it.

"So anyway back to the ward move saga" I encouraged.

She responded in an equally light tone. "Well as I was saying it got to the stage where it was me or arse grabbing scary drama teacher that had to go. I was blissfully unaware of the full extend of her obsession with me other than she wanted my arse for Christmas, birthday well everyday really. Yes I was getting pissed off and the stronger I grew the more pissed off I got. She stalked me when I was looking and properly more so when I wasn't. It was around the same time as one of the nurses had a chunk bitten out of her thigh. Proper big bite it was. Not sure which one of the crazies was responsible for it but what was clear was that they stayed in the locked room and had the window bit covered up for days. It was also during the period that pretend nurse Gwen thought my friend who came sometimes was a lizard. It didn't help matters that Haber (that's what we called her down the pub) was playing along with the whole lizard thing and when my back was turned she was down on the floor doing a reptile like movement with her tongue. Gwen loved it; Haber loved it properly for very different reasons, Haber's all too often sexual. When she visited Haber had also made another friend. Marcus...he looked like Jesus and didn't speak, only in a very garbled quiet way. What was cool was that as soon as Haber heard his voice she replied to him in German. Her mum was German, didn't look like Jesus but did only ever use German to communicate. So that's how come Haber was fluent and able to help Marcus. Scary but no one else had realised it was actually proper talk just not English. He left pretty soon after that.

I know I go off the subject but I'm trying to give you a flavour of the stuff that was going on at the same time as the ward move thing. So my stuff was gathered and I was hurried away to the opposite ward across a balcony corridor only the brave would explore. I hated it that I was somewhere different with a new set of scary ill people to stare at me. This ward (the new one) was home to Randall. I met him as he was dragged into the locked up room, the whole set up was a mirror image of my previous dwelling so the lock up was too in the big open corridor with lots of doors off it. Randall had just punched a shrink full in the face and given him a real shiner. I quite liked Randall, he still had spirit. He spent his time in the cell waving through the window, happy I think that he had managed to air his anger despite the present consequence.

Margaret was also an interesting demonstration of life on the ward. She was far too busy to sit down to eat, and she only drank on the move. She was full of energy and mischievous like a child with cute cheeks. She spent her days organising the pictures on the wall. In Margaret's world they were all the wrong way up until she painlessly went round turning each picture on its head, of which there were many. All of similar theme colour and lack of interest, the hospital seemed to house anything of retired value from people's homes. Margaret upped her game at one point of her stay and stole all the pictures off the walls and then hid them along with some other treasures that she had accumulated, all not fitting in to her scenery. I thought she was fab. They called her manic, I didn't know why but to me she was a genius and so much fun. She had medicine to stop her turning the pictures the other way and stealing her treasures. It worked, Margaret stopped doing the picture thing but she stopped smiling to. She didn't even wear her smile when she left.

So most of the days the ward had its own in house entertainment. There were a couple of lovely people who worked the night shift. I didn't bother them and in turn they didn't bother me. One of the ladies used to make hot drinks when the patients were going to bed. I liked her a lot; she spoke to me like I wasn't invisible which made me feel alive.

I wasn't allowed to go back to the other ward at all which was harsh as I had made friends with some people to make the day pass by. Nobody told me why which made it difficult for me to understand but now it makes more sense. Then it made me cross. I knew that arse catcher was the reason for my departure which pissed me off. The more I thought about it the more pissed off I felt. For all the groping and letching and touching near the privacy of my pants they had done nothing. She was relentless in her mission and the staff seemed to acknowledge little of her behaviour toward me. Plus now I'd got shipped out for her trouble. I didn't know how long I had to stay in the hospital. I was told that they were waiting for a place for me in a detox unit. Hospital workers hold no responsibility for time when delivering that type of news. You say....how long? They answer with silence. So I'd got myself proper cross and bored about the whole move thing. What was I to do about my crossness? That was easy...I was going to shift my teenage arse over to freaky drama teacher and pop her one. The simplicity of a world where the rules seem to change without warning".

"You hit her?" I was surprised by the twist in her jackanory what's the story tale.

"Patience my friend I'm getting to the bit about hitting…I went marching over the balcony corridor donning my innocent bravery and through the double doors of the ward. I marched at pace down the corridor with many rooms and past the nursing station on my right. I was at the time unaware I had drawn an almost Pied Piper following behind me. Scanning as I paced I couldn't see my arse catcher opponent and so I continued through more doors and downwards toward the dormitory where in the distance I could see her through the glass door protecting her. My pace quickened, as did the steps behind me, when I realised the war drum thrumbing behind me was people it was too late. Their approach had been calculated and mine had been naive. I touched the glass door before I felt hands on me. It was however as close as I got on that occasion, she would keep for another day but for now I was terrified as to what was happening to me."

"What do you mean?" I asked, I was confused by comedy girl's sudden change in the story map. "What was happening to you? Had you hurt your self?" again I could tell that the next chapter would hold meaning to her journey stronger than other more amusing excerpts.

"No I didn't hurt myself. It was the hands of plenty that I had felt on me stopping my entry through the glass door (we both looked up having an almost 'Charlie and the glass elevator' moment but not quite so appropriate for the humour to slip in which always made it more funny). The hands were rough and assertive and as I turned to see who their owner was I was welcomed by three then four staff members all looking surprisingly like guards at this time. They were grabbing and pulling at me, one female I think or an unfortunate gender mix up man mistake."

"God what did you do?" I was tense for the moment, feeling nervous for comedy girl's reply.

"Fight or flight kicked in and I've never been one for the air so I returned with force. I was quite a strong little thing, really solid.... I think some people refer to it as fat! You probably can't imagine me chunky..."

"Oh I think I can" I responded silently having had the chunky meet and greet comedy wave owner I first was graced with at the start of this epic conversation.... but I replied with my eyes.

"Maybe you can" she continued. "I had done martial arts from the start of my double figure years and was a bit of a dab hand at it. Id always trained with the adults and mostly men due to my apparently unnatural strength for a child. My parents had first been drawn to this when they had popped into my primary school to ask the teacher if they could crush the bullying comments that the girls used to throw at me. I didn't mind them, wasn't bothered but my dad was a little concerned that I would retaliate at some point. I was like a sponge that soaked it all up but as with anything I suppose sometimes there is no more room to soak. The teacher had responded with practised conversation and done little to act on my parents' concern. That was until months later they were called in again to discuss just how I had managed to pick up one of the larger boys and hold him laying flat above my head in my arms which were straight.... just like I'd watched the strong men do on the telly. The teacher was most concerned at the shock absorbed by the dinnerlady. I always remember her face, it was full up of years of powder foundation and heavy lipstick.

She had to go home early from her duties as she couldn't quite believe that she had witnessed a child holding another child up in the air waiting for what may happen next. As my punishment I would always have opted for the school's decision, a cane becoming my welcomed friend in my early years. On this occasion my Dad in his strictness questioned me about the incident and I proudly told him that I held the boy up above me until he said sorry. What would you have done if he hadn't said sorry was my fathers question, with which he was sure of the answer I gave. Id have thrown him away dad.

After that there was another tale that my father used to amuse other grown ups with. It was during a weekend I was away in the caravan with my dad. No one else just me and my dad. They were the best times the world ever had to offer. We were getting ready to go home after a fun weekend. My dad full up of Budweiser with American ring pulls and me full up of brown ale.... Always allowed a four pack on our weekends. Dad had some trouble doing all the heavy bits as often his asthma kept him company with such demand. I used to run around doing the busy bits and dad would reverse the car on target for the caravan to land on. I stood directing him by the front guiding wheel of the caravan and with my left hand waved the direction he needed to take. With marked procession I gave the thumbs up for him to cease his manoeuvres. He shut the car door and walked round to where I was standing. He greeted me with surprised eyes as I stood my right hand firmly clasping the handle infront of the guide wheel pole. I was holding the caravan full off the ground with its back end almost tickling the grass. The car tow bar was directly underneath. Can I put it on now dad? He replied laughing....yes the idea is that you wind the wheel up to hold the weight of the van Donks (his tireless name for me) and then unwind it down. It was years before I realised my part in that story.

So anyway strength had always joined me in my growing up years and these heavy hands needed to get off. I fought back!! As hard as I could. Funny really 'cos I had never really fought with anyone aside from my sister where face punching was barred (the unwritten rule we had). I had got a good ole fashioned kicking once. Now that was a story. I had been out on the town with a new girl at the hostel. She had come from South Africa, to stay for a while not just for the evening. We were chasing the shots around town and after 16 we felt it was time to go home. We stopped for one last one in the pub close to the hostel, as a night cap. We were about to leave when I clocked a girl who about 6 months previously had given me a pasting on the bus as I travelled home late at night. Didn't know her, she just started to hit me. I, at the time never thought to fight back. So anyway here she was in front of me. She was sat with a large group of equally scary looking birds and one boy. I went up to her. (oh how simple everything seems when you are draped in confidence that vodka brings). I asked her why she had hit me. I then asked her not to do it again. All very polite."

I stared at comedy girl…."yeah I know" she replied "but it made sense at the time", She continued " so anyway she got all bolshy in front of her ugly friends and said she may do it to me again one day. I went to walk away, she laughed at me. I turned and back handed her full in the face. I knew it was a direct hit because her legs went up in the air cartoon style and she flew back on her chair landing chair back to the floor but still in the seated position. Oops I thought to myself in my drunken mind. That worked! I turned to the exit and ran. I was in big trouble. The pub entrance had stone steps leading down to ground level. I was at the top of those steps when ugly birds caught me. I got to the bottom of them by being thrown down them. I was grateful for the pain relief so often gained from being wasted. Still on the floor I got kicked and punched. A police van stopped. The ugly ones said I was their very drunk friend and that they were trying to get me off the floor to take me home. The police van left. As they did high five slapping to each other in response to their quick thinking I grabbed the chance and ran. I only reached a side alley before the mob caught up. I shouted to my South African new friend to run. (I was hoping she would get a little help, she never returned.). I was knocked to the floor and given a beating. The boy had joined in. Eventually they left me. My clothes were ripped and my face doing 'tom and jerry' throbbing. Dragged my arse back to the hostel where the beast was waiting with open door. The beast was what we called the warden woman. One of three who always thought she should be the most senior. It grated on her that she was not. Anyway me and the beast had not got on since I moved there. She liked the boys better. The boys, and the girls with no spirit. The beast shouted at me to get to my room. I went to the bathroom area to wash my face and clean myself up. The South African was sitting in the shower folding socks. She didn't look up....that in itself was random. My head and my eye were cut, my lip was cut but most impressively I had a full boot print on the side of my face reaching right round to my ear. This got blacker as the night turned in to day. The beast never asked if I was ok. She was hard like slate. So anyway back to the story...

I struggled and pushed and by all accounts was quite a handful I think. Reinforcement's came and I was put to the floor."

Welcome to My World

"Did you hit anyone?" I asked, as I wasn't sure what the fight back entailed

"No no hitting just trying to get them off me. By the time I was put to the floor there was a handful of men laying on and all around me and one woman doing a 'I don't know quite where to put myself' dance. It was horrible. I'd been taken completely off the ground with my legs jammed together my head and arms all wrapped up. When I got to the ground my struggle continued I just wanted them off me and I didn't know why they were on me in the first place. I was scared I was going for that treatment thing I had watched posh lady be taken to. It's how they seemed to take people and I didn't want to go. I was so trapped. Do you know if your putting your arm in your jumper or your sock on and suddenly you cant push any further or move yourself and for a minute a wave of panic sets in? Well imagine that feel but with a hole sunarmi of panic waves rather than the little teaser accompanying the sock trap manoevre. Eventually I got tired of fighting, for a minute I relaxed my German shot putter arms. As I did so I felt room to move.... So I did. I was up from the floor and running like the wind down to the front of the ward double door place. My opponents were quick to chase. I just wanted out of there, I didn't want any of the electrical shocks or what ever else was past the doors down the corridor that no one ever spoke about. As I got to the door I was pulled away. I asked them to let go to get off me to leave me alone. I wanted to walk outside or anything just not be near the hospital guards. The fight continued but with me playing a part little in comparison. I wasn't fighting anymore. I just wanted them off now. I kept asking but to deaf ears. Again I was thrown to the floor. The nurse who had done the awkward 'find a job to do' dance previously was now sort of shouting at me.

They called it 'section', they said it was for my own good. They said I couldn't go anywhere and that a doctor was coming. I had no idea what was going on. I felt scared inside and trapped. Normally when you get cross you can walk it off. She said she thought I was going to the pub...how random was that in my head. Why would I be going to the pub I'd spent the last 5 or 6 weeks of my life trying to stop that part of my life consuming my world? It was a crazy time and I was locked out of the things that work for me. So the doctor came and asked me questions and then I was able to go for a walk after which I returned to my new ward again. It was kind of odd really and left me with fear of what can happen in the caring place that was my temporary home. The nurse came and said it was no longer 'section' what ever that meant.

Chapter Five

By now I was beginning to realise I needed to learn the rules quick and so I began to ask few but important questions. Firstly about section. I had noticed a few people had it. So one of them who was quite young and ok to talk to I asked what it meant. When I understood it felt more scary!"

I was fully aware of what comedy girl was describing. We used it at work.... It being Mental health law. The power to hold someone against their will. What had happened to her was a nurse's holding power. I'd had to use it only once but with heart breaking guilt and the belief that it was for the greater good. She knew I knew...we didn't need to confirm this.

"So" I questioned "was that the end of the drama bird saga?"

"Not quite "she replied (oh how I love a twist) "there was one more occasion, it was much later on just before I left for my next adventure. Scary drama bird had been moved, interestingly, to the ward where I was. I had grown in confidence and was now quite savvy to the laws and rules of the place. As soon as she arrived she recognised me as her prey from previous weeks. The stalking began and with an air of anticipation I bided my time. It was afternoon and I was sitting in the long corridor room by the window. She took her perch close enough for me to hear her waterfall of comments that preceeded her arrival. Your mother this, your mother that bla bla bla...for a while I listened and then with a spring in my step not unlike the approach to the 'horse' the gymnasts use I pounced. I was over the table that separated our fighting arena in seconds. I grabbed her by the collar and with the grace of an open cape I floated her back across the table and up against the wall. My arms fully stretched helped me to realise she was slightly taller than I had guesstimated in my role-playing mind. She was huge and just a little bit cross to say the least. Having come to the very quick decision that I had bitten off more than I could chew it was confirmed when I found that during my initial floating attack I had caught up her necklace in my grasp and this was now in jigsaw pieces falling from my hand around her collar. I was in big huge trouble with scary drama bird far bigger and strong and angrier than me. What a plonker I was anticipating a large kicking that through my error I should deserve. Fortunately for me the guards were approaching, just as they had done all those weeks previously. Only this time I was so pleased to see them. As I stood back and watched the finish of what I had started I witnessed her at full force as did the larger than life full team of men 6 or 7 that were man handling her to the lock up where she stayed for a while. The only guilt I felt was that the guards had fought my battle. I had received weeks of her garbage and groping and dirty talk. I was full up.

That night it was the first time I ever asked a nurse if I could have some medicine. It was the only time too. One thing about the relationship I had formed with the nurse workers was that if I asked for something it was for real. The nurse on duty that night battled for what seemed like hours with some faceless doctor on the phone who insisted he knew me better having never met or heard my name. The night nurse and me had a chat. I told her one day I was going to be a nurse. She said she hoped one day I was. I meant it. I never said stuff I didn't mean...why would you? That night I had some medicine it was the stuff that made my nose do the underwater forward roll thing. That night it helped!"

It seemed comedy girl had a story for everything, or maybe that's just how she had coped with the memories that could all too easily drag you down. Some of her tales had an air of bitch to them. Maybe it was the adolescent ways that feel the whole world is wrong. I portrayed to her that her stories were interesting and full of description. That her world then was broken down into daily diaries of the mental hospital. I asked her…."When did it stop"

"Not for a while" she replied, "why, do you have to leave?" It was the first time she had given me room to escape properly. But the truth was I had no better place to be than to listen and learn from someone else's episodes in life.

She could see I made no attempt to move and so with a cheeky grin she continued. "My most comical encounter is one I must share" her eyes were laughing as she spoke, the comedy flowing in giggle river, I was poised for her next tale.

"On the ward the new but not so new now ward I was privileged to share a dormitory with a rather demanding lady called Rose.   Rose was from the Caribbean originally and her Jamaican twang still laced her voice. She was a comfortably rounded lady as wide as she was tall. Her voice deep and controlling and her needs much the same. She or one of the nurses would order me down to the shop where I would have to buy Rose's snuff. I wasn't arguing with her and so often trotted down and back with the purchase. I used to be woken up at night by a running water noise. This was Rose peeing in some make shift potty she stored under the bed secret from the staff. Funny really as I think the whole dorm was too scared to reveal her secret, we just all lay awake listening to her pee night after night.

Rose could become a bit over friendly sometimes and break in to people's personal space. She would say very loudly whilst approaching her victim (of which there were many) Baby, Baby come to Mama. Her arms wide open to the fearful recipient. She would then continue her calls like a bird calling to her young. Baby come to Mama. When no movement was made towards her she would change her slant slightly. If baby won't come to Mama,........ Mama come to baby. At which point she would entomb the person her target into her arms and large bosom until Rose decided to let go. It was fun to watch as long as you were not a part of her show.

The young one who I had become chatting buddies with was watching TV one evening when Rose spied her for the bosom. She began with her Baby come to Mama routine and so on. The young one looked at me, I was already laughing, as I knew what was coming. Rose launched herself at the young one and her cheek was fixed firmly to Rose's bosom as she straddled the chair. The young one's eyes told me to run and get help. I was so busy pissing my pants laughing hard that I took a bit longer than maybe she had wished. The nurses came and with a tug of war type system they detached Rose from the young one's cheek. She was cross that I had taken so long to get help. I was however unaffected by her crossness, still doing belly laughing. She got pay back.... Big time!

One morning I was rudely awoken by firstly the huge struggle I had to breathe. I was really scared; the young one, also in the dorm, was sleeping across the room, which seemed a mile away from where I needed her to be. I was scared to open my eyes as the fight for breath was overpowering. And then I heard the unwelcome commentary that accompanied my trauma like no other...Baby won't come to Mama, Mama come to

Welcome to My World

Baby. My eyes pinged open and in front of my eyelid curtains was the star of the show. Rose in all her bed time glory was laying face down from head to toe on top of me. My breathing restriction experience was Rose compressing my chest all ten hundred tons of her. She was trying to move her self upwould so that my lips greeted her unsecured bosom. This was never going to be fun. I couldn't move Rose 'cos it really was hard to breath. The commotion had woken the rest of the dorm and the young one, although pausing for at least some poetic justice, ran to get the human 'Rose' crane that the now practiced staff formed.   They came, they shouted, they looked and then they helped. The relief I felt was unimaginable…I'd been 'Rosed' and with the greatest of power."

I was laughing out loud with comedy girl by my side. The image she had conjured up was, I trust, very close to the truth and with little left to the imagination. In my work I had met some fascinating people with some unfortunate symptoms that accompany mental illness.

I pondered on my experiences sharing with my companion a moment that amused me when I visited that memory. The patient was a real live wire. She was only about four-foot tall but with a mastermind of attacks. I thought she was great. Difficult but great. Her days on the ward were made up of chain link attacks on each person who got in her way. She was relentless and as you broke her grasp on one person the next victim takes their place. I was discussing what we could do to perhaps manage her behaviour with the psychiatrist who graced us very rarely. He sat on the office chair and I squatted down as I did so often in place of other,s favoured seating choices.   I was explaining that she was becoming increasingly difficult to manage with the tools we had on offer when, as if on cue, she launched herself at me and more directly my hair. With artistic precision she immediately twisted and then pulled. A now practised act we had all been privy to. My head was now pinned to the floor as her mouth began biting and her free hand began the nails down face drag. I was so engrossed in my quest to find the answer with the psychiatrist I simply carried on my conversation from my floor position. My lack of reaction showed I was not the best multi-tasker and that I could only manage one thing at a time. The comical value of that experience allows my colleagues to refer to it so very often.

I wondered if comedy girl had saturated her memory of stories when she broke my thoughts. "So the next thing was the detox rehab adventure."

She was reaching in her over size satchel bag that had come in with her as she entered the coffeehouse (see I'm still jazzing up my venue). Comedy girl with the lesser hips pulled out some papers all tied together with one of those green string things with metal ends you had to use quite unsuccessfully at school. The paper edges were curled similar to an outgrown perm and coffee marked its used history. She looked at me and then handed the papers over. With confusion I asked what it was. She replied "it's the rehab road, I wondered if you fancied reading it. When I returned I wrote down whatever I could.... like a story. I didn't finish it but the words are from a teenager and seen through innocentish eyes. You don't have to but that story I don't want to spoil with my matured knowledge. This is how I thought it was at the time. No charades or underlining motivation. Just me telling me what happened. I've scrubbed the names out though…some things are just private. I called it 'the hardest part of life is growing up'"

Welcome to My World

The irony was I really believed that statement to be true until as an adult you realise you watch people spending their whole life chasing those times. I took hold of the story to which I was keen to be introduced. "Shall I read it now?" I questioned. She looked out of the window and so my eyes fell silent and I began to read...

Chapter Six

The hardest part of life is growing up by Jodie Lee aged 17 and a half. Who was Jodie Lee I thought? Anyway I continued.....

"Take it easy" they shouted from a distance. I could barely hear it over the loud and monotonous drone of the train struggling away from the platform. I was left on my own. Strangers looking into my eyes. I tried continuously to dodge their stares but each time I managed to break away from one glare another was ready to take over. Do all these people know where I was going and for what reason? Surely not. But it felt that way. Suddenly I was startled by a sharp tap on my left shoulder. It was my old friend Paranoia who invited himself to accompany me for the whole of my adventure journey. Over the loudspeaker came the all to threatening list of items offered in the buffet car. " hot and cold beverages including beer, wine and spirits" just what I didn't want or need to hear.

I knew if I had an alcoholic drink all my fears would disappear. I also knew that I would then be back on the road of being an active alcoholic. What a choice!

With paranoia sitting by my side and the continual thought of there being alcohol within reach hanging over my head the first stage of my trip was not in the least bit pleasant.

My eyes began to swell. The imaginary lump appeared in my throat which made it difficult for me to swallow. Cry? How could I cry in front of all these people. The tears began to develop within the rims of my eyes to the extent of overflowing. Singlely at first they travelled down my cheeks rebounding and then falling only to be lost in the material which made up my sweater. I tried to stop this most common but embarrassing reaction to 'leaving my friends' but the more I fought it the worst I became. My face beginning to spring into numerous different shapes which must have looked comical. Fighting back tears is a losing battle, you may as well sit and let it all flood out, which eventually I realised.

"The train is now arriving in London where it will terminate. Could all passengers kindly remove all their belongs from the train and make their way on to platform 15 thank you"

What was I going to do now? I hadn't got a bloody clue, all I could think about was how much easier it would be to travel down those extremely steep and seemingly everlasting escalators which led toward the tube station with a couple of whiskies or G 'n' Ts inside of me. I didn't have much time to catch my next train which departed from one of the other stations heading for Westwood. It was a battle on the tube at the best of times but without my security and courage I found in a short it was near impossible.

As I understood I could travel the whole distance with this one ticket I held in my hand. All I needed was some cocky machine which was going to eat it or any other unthinkable disaster.

Even though I walked slowly the escalator was, I'm sure, travelling toward me. I had panic attacks on the ones in Debenhams and those were like babies compared with this monster who was about to attack me and my three holdalls wrapped untidily around my neck and of course not forgetting the extra weight of paranoia on my shoulders....

....I was on! My eyes shut so tightly it felt like the lids had been stapled together. My knees knocking like a one man band. Before I'd left everyone had said to me "In London act like a Londoner would. Be cool, be carefree and most of all be confident." I had failed at this miserably. I could so easily have been mistaken for a constipated Japanese art student with a shop's range of camera attached to all parts of my body. Who could have asked for a better start!

Once on the tube it was no problem. I was rather restricted with my bags and so found it much easier to stand. My stop was the first so I had prepared for alighting almost immediately after hoping on. One thing I did know was that the underground trains' automatic doors found it hilarious to trap you between them. It would have been ok if I was an anorexic banana but as it was me a 10 and half stone slightly roly poly healthy young woman. I was not to be caught out I found getting on and off the tube compared well with the dance the hokey cokey.

At the tube station there was a wonderful device called the walkalater. It was easy to get the hang of, you just walked on the machine, sort of like a moving hill and it did the rest for you. In fact I class myself as a bit of a professional on this device and after my third time round I developed the skill of walking as you went. It was wonderful. You seemed to travel at such a speed. My hair flowed and I felt like the lady clinging to Tom Cruise on his motorbike in Top Gun (of course I had the looks to match).

At the station where the train was heading for Westwood there was just one more monster and then none for a while. I was feeling pretty confident, not safe, just confident. Until the man behind me on the escalator pointed out that the queue which preceeded him was not people just enjoying the ride but waiting for me to move my "fat arse" onto the other side as this was the side for the professionals. Those bolshy business men who like to wear their blakeys down by running on the escalators. He continued that I should have read the signs saying 'stand to the right'. Of course I could not alternate sides. I couldn't even move! My reply was simply "sorry but I'm not budging" In a more choice use of grammar naturally!

I was knackered and glad to sit down at station. I'd made good time and had about half an hour before my next train departed. Time enough for a sandwich and a couple of fags. I'm sure my nose had built in beer sensors because after parking my bum and unloading the bags I looked up only to see that directly opposite me was the station's very own Off Licence.....'How Quaint'. Again I subsided my cravings. For the sole reason that I was going to a drug and alcohol rehabilitation centre for 18 months to get sorted out. My friends deserved more than I had been offering.

On the train to Westwood I sat at the same table as a man and woman travelling back from a course as far as I could gather from the information relayed through my hearing aid, which just conveniently slipped up to full volume, not that I'd ever dream of eavesdropping. They actually came across more than adequately friendly toward each other. My imagination being somewhat over sufficient began to concoct all sorts of excuses they had been using to their independent partners for, at a rough guess, the last 7 months. It was almost sickly to see the early thirties woman with, I estimate, 2 young children, 5 and 7, fall contently to sleep on the more later thirties gent pretending to be early twenties. Mills and Boom readers would have had a field day.

Its amazing how time flies when you're having fun. My connect train was already waiting at Westwood Station so I did a rather undignified wonder-woman sprint across platforms to leap onto the old style train with no connecting carriages and doors on each one. Only I could pick the carriage with a oldish man sat cross-legged bent as a broom handle, a man so pissed up I was quite content on just inhaling the fumes. The carriage also had a 'would be' punk rocker. All my type of people!

I felt bored of travelling now. I felt fed up, worn out and just sat day dreaming of my pillow. Sharfield was only a short distance away from Westwood but it dragged out. I've never seen such a farty station apart from the one at the local village near where I lived. Nothing tops that. "Welcome to Sharfield" was the only instruction given over the intercom. Where was the red carpet? Didn't they know Royalty was coming? Well me which was the next best thing. What a bloody welcome I had just travelled half way across the country to some shitty place in the middle of nowhere and there wasn't even somebody to meet me. I was in a bit of a mess really . I had no idea which direction to head in. All I knew was I had to be at Sharfield probation office at 2:00pm. I spared no expense (I hadn't really a choice). I hailed a taxi and away we went. He must have recognised I was not from the area and insisted it would be quicker to get from the station to the centre of town if we travelled by the motorway. God did I look that gullible? Being in no mood for an argument with my first encounter of the inhabitants of such out of touch place I paid the ridiculous fair and got out. 1:40pm, 20 minutes to waste and a pub in sight. The rain was knocking on my head, it felt that my skin was no longer porous and I was now completely saturated inside out. I began to cry again, what the hell. My street 'cred' had been reduced to just about zero anyway standing outside the probation office. How much harm could a few tears of nerves and sadness combined do? After all I deserved it. Id made the journey, not had a drink and continually achieved only limited conversation with paranoia. If that didn't allow me a bit of 'I want to feel sorry for myself 'time, what did?

I'd been waiting 40 minutes and then in she waltzed. Rather than just a plain 'hello Heather' from the receptionist I felt a fanfare to be more apt. Still she did not acknowledge I was there. If this was a typical Sharfield woman I didn't want to know. Stuck up bitch. Eventually she came and introduced herself as "Ms Heather Bumstead" . I couldn't help thinking how appropriate it was. Her rear was so enormous that if she bent over astronomers would probably record it as an eclipse. In a way I felt sorry for her. She was really unlucky. Her hair was obviously greying rapidly and her attempt to disguise the fact with rather unprofessional highlights had failed. Make up wasn't her strong point either, with summer bronze blusher plastered half way up her ears and apple rose lipstick mistakenly placed on her teeth she could only be classed as far from attractive. I shouldn't imagine she was much under forty although she constantly chewed gum like a teenager, which I objected to, and made no secret of the fact. Tactfully suggesting that she'd just given up smoking and it was noticeable. It would be no exaggeration to say that we didn't hit it off. She gestured me to follow her up the stairs. I obliged but lagged behind if only to keep a distance from her hips which swayed dangerously far in her 'lets try and be modern' A-line skirt. The shoes topped off this not very fetching summer number and really the only word to describe them was...Navy. Should I leave now or later?

Although the office where we sat had 'no smoking' signs plastered every where I still enquired whether I could. The answer was not unexpected and instead I fidgeted annoyingly with my coat zip.

"So you want to join us at Brenten house is that right?" of course it was bloody right what else did she think I was doing there...sight-seeing?

"Yes" I replied a bit to innocent for words. "What drugs were you on – a heroin junkie, acid, Thames?"
Oh she was in with the words. Drugs for goodness sake. What was I doing here I wasn't a junkie far from, anyway needles made me woozy. I knew the place was a combined drink/drugs rehab but I was under the impression it would be slightly more tame. Oh shit! Maybe I could soften her with a witty comment like paracetamol....maybe not!

Heather's 'I'm doing you a favour and you'd better remember it' attitude was I found, extremely patronising. I had received no information about Brenten house previous to my interview and so everything I was now hearing was new. It sounded all most comical. The way she was explaining it to me. I later found out she was not exaggerating and was totally serious about the 1 or 2 rules she had briefly mentioned. No sex, no swearing, no jewellery, no make-up, no freedom.

My suspicions became firm when she asked me to sign some forms. Stressing that a mark would be adequate if I couldn't write. Who the hell was this woman, questioning my intelligence? Heather Bumstead obviously hadn't had the courtesy to read up on who she was interviewing. She didn't know why I was there, what I was 'on' and although I'd hand written my application, whether I could read or write. She was certainly good material for the school of learning respect.

"Its tough at Brenten , do you think you can complete the program?"

How could I possibly know that. All I had was a 5 minute undetailed description of the place. No mention of the programme whatsoever. I wanted to run but I had to say yes, if only to annoy Ms Heather Bumstead, the gum-chewing geriatric.

It was just what she didn't want to hear..."are you sure?". I could see her face cringe at the thought of all the paperwork she would have to complete. The numerous forms to return to the DSS for the most important reason...the money. The damage it would do to her rather squarely shaped false nails. Tragic! With a quick flutter of my eye lashes (it worked for Brook Shields) I confidently replied "well I'd like to try."

At the time I didn't understand why she would not let me leave her side from then on. I'd asked to get fags and chocolate. The answer was a short sharp army instruction of "NO".

"Put your stuff in the boot". I expected her to drive a Sierra ghia. What stood in front of me was a hairdryer on wheels. The latest Peugeot 205, very expensive but that's about it. Where was the boot on these things? As we drove in complete silence I had the chance to survey my new surroundings. I wouldn't have thought it possible to reach such rural surroundings in ten minutes but in this nippy vehicle we managed. Heather's driving skills were also against her. I'd never seen so much grass. There were hills everywhere. Trees which were pruned to the same design as a hair style a teacher at my school used to model. Sort of pear shaped. All types of farm animals roamed freely across the fields. Where was Sainsburys and Marks and Sparks? The sign welcoming you to Croxet went past like a shooting star at the speed we were travelling. I got the general idea Ms Bumstead was in a hurry to dump me off. The indicator went down to left, we braked. After peeling my nose and lips off the windscreen I saw it...Brenten House. It was how I'd always imagined the old house of James' Aunt in James and the giant peach...Ugly. I bailed out of the car (took off the parachute pack she had equipped me with, just in case) and approached the front door. Countless pairs of eyes stared at me through all windows of the house. It was like being marooned on a desert island. I could feel my self looking rather unattractive as I entered the house, but who wouldn't after 4 1/2 hours of solid travelling half of which was through London and its famous smog. The eyes followed me and became features of figures which faintly resembled people. I had the same feeling as my first day at a new school. A classroom full of kids all curious to know who I was, where I was from, basically everything about you. They all looked so scruffy and tired. Where were all the staff? Were there any?

My thoughts were broken into by Heather's familiar drone. "this is the new girl (god it rang through my ears) she's come to join us. An embarrassed grin sprang to my face. I felt really stupid. I was still clutching my three hold-alls. It's easy to imagine just how pathetic I looked.

Two women came towards me looking similar to each other. Both with unattended hair and very drawn out faces. Heather introduced us. This is Bonnie and this is Susan...My dignity was lost during the search I had to succumb to.

Welcome to My World

"These two girls will be looking after you" were the last words of Ms 'I'm better than the rest of you' Bumstead and so I was left alone.

In front of me stood two 'girls' (I wouldn't have shared the same choice in vocabulary, they were both 30+). Fashion obviously not one of their strong points, skin tight, stretch jeans (the extra stretch was certainly not wasted) with holes at the knees. T-shirts and pumps, none of which were clean. Staff or residents? I hadn't a bloody clue.

I was taken in to the annex. A pool table took up most of this small room. At least there must be some form of civilization if nothing else. I assumed I'd still be able to shoot pool. My favourite pastime, often a sign of misspent youth it was said.

All the curious eyes had disappeared now. I was left with Bonnie and Susan. Across the room was another new chap, his face looking bewildered and scared, much the same as I imagined mine to be. He'd also got someone with him who was kitted out in glad rags. I began to wonder whether in was meant to be therapeutic. Wearing scruffy clothes?

"Have you bought any drugs in with you?"
"No" I replied slightly taken aback. So it was assumed I was a user.
"Well we'll have to search you anyway. It's the rules" Bonnie explained.

Wasn't my word good enough? I think they felt like Cagney and Lacey in a stake out. I wasn't too sure of what they meant 'search me'. My imagination stepped up to full power. If you were suspected of drug trafficking at airports you were taken to a little room and while continually being patronised made to strip naked and searched inside and out. That's what I'd heard. No lawyer, nothing. Where was the room? My eyes scanned each partition for secret doors or such like. Panic set in…how could I strip? I'd got my period.

"What do you mean search me?" Directing the question at Bonnie. She came across more in charge.
"Don't worry, we both had to go through it, anyway we're all girls together. That didn't answer my bloody question.

All my jewellery was taken away. That upset me. Before I left Remi, one of closest friends had pointed to his ring that I had been wearing on my finger for the past year and said "when you get lonely or you feel like giving up, look at the ring and I'll be with you"; fat chance of that now. After much protest I deposited it in the open brown envelop. Bonnie said that in Brenten, everyone starts off alike. It would be no good some people walking around with the equivalent of the crown jewels and others who weren't so fortunate with nothing. Although their actions were justified it made the instruction no less unpleasant. Susan was in charge of recording all my possessions. In her left hand she held a tatty clipboard and in her right, a disposable Bic roller pen. I felt she'd be more suited participating in a survey usually situated outside of Debenhams. It had been my policy to ignore that type of person. If only I could do that now.

After taking away my walkman, tapes, writing paper, cigarette lighters, address, money and just about everything else I'd brought along with me Bonnie suggested we moved upstairs to our bedroom. With the extra emphasis on the 'our'. I assumed this was not going to be in the same category as a honeymoon suite at the Ritz. And that I was possibly going to be sharing with these other two 'spring chickens'. As I gazed into the open door of something much similar to the shape of a semi-detached cardboard box I wanted to stand to attention. A friend from the town where I lived had spent three years in the army and up until now I had trouble imagining the living conditions. The floor in this dorm was so clean you could have eaten off it. The beds were made to perfection. It was hard to think somebody ruined their appearance by sleeping in them. The standards were 100% which made the dorm far from homely. How could such scruffy people live in such perfection? Where was the sock left for days on the temperature gauge of the radiator? And the clothes taken off from the night before, usually found decorating the wardrobe door or a corner chair. The place was spotless. No dust, no rubbish in the bin and most importantly, no mess.

A set of bunks beds faced the entrance and to the right was a single bed. "Please let me not be on the top bunk" I repeated the request in my mind. The reason being that since I can remember I've always had a tendency to fall out of bed and carry on sleeping. In hospital the staff had found this a sort of highlight of an evening and quite comical. But a bunk bed six feet off the ground. We could be in serious trouble. To my relief the lower bed was unmade and I was instructed that in fact that would mine.

With in minutes the floor was covered with the contents of my three hold-alls which Susan and Bonnie began to search. Slap bang in the middle of the chaos was the pile of Tampax I had hastily packed. My face began to turn hot and the uneasy feeling of embarrassment rushed through me. With an unsure laugh I questioned my own action of not putting them in a bag or something. Their response was only to inform me that tampax were something supplied as and when required free of charge…some perk!

Although Bonnie and Sue were residents (I wouldn't be put in a room with two staff) there was a certain air of authority about them. They made me feel so small. It may of course been paranoia reminding me it was still around.

The search was not as bad as my expectations but still left me feeling I had absolutely no privacy left. This was true. All my personal things which I chose usually not to show people had been looked through. My folder, a taboo property as my friends named it, was taken away. Any clothes that were a bit fancy joined the rest of my things later taken to the property shed. Along with all my personal things I had brought along an aerosol deodorant (ozone friendly). Why the bloody hell wasn't I allowed to keep that? "The rules" Bonnie stated (she was good at avoiding questions.).

It was now becoming obvious why all the people I'd seen on my way in looked so scruffy. How could they attempt to keep tidy with none of what I'd class as essentials. This place was crazy.

Towards the end of the search Bonnie and Sue advised me as to some of the ways of the house. Minutes later the conversation strayed on to life stories. Bonnie, who'd be there the longer time of 6 months wasn't really very talkative. I was grateful as the thought of what to say to a 37 year old Heroin junkie currently fighting her ex-husband in the courts for custody of her two kids was scary. On the other hand Sue wasn't so shy. At the end of the conversation I was toying with the idea of changing my name to Aunt Clare Rayner or Marj

Proops. One of her troubles in early teens was the fact she became anorexic. At first I thought it was a joke but when I laughed and saw that nobody else was laughing I realised she was serious. It was difficult to believe that the 'not so slim' figure in front of me with spare tyres enough to supply Ford Car company until year x had suffered anorexia nervosa, a sometimes fatal disease. She was obviously well on the road to a full recovery.

I couldn't help noticing that both Bonnie and Sue had the most manly shaped arms and hands. Sue's were worst. Her fingers reminded me of the individually wrapped cigars Jimmy Saville smokes. They were enormous. I'm not really sure whether it was a natural deformity or a reaction caused by heroin. If that's possible? It seemed too much of a coincidence that Bonnie also had the same arm structure.

"Right then we better get back to work". The instruction came from Bonnie. Sue 'fat fingers' agreed.

Work? What were they on about. I was beginning to think I'd come to the wrong place (deep down I know this was impossible with Ms Bumstead as escort). This was a Drug Rehabilitation centre wasn't it? Not a remand home. Jesus I knew I done something wrong by becoming an alcoholic but I didn't realise the sentence was going to be this steep. Where was all the one to one counselling I'd seen on the telly? Come to that where were all the staff? I thought it would be the policy when a new resident came to automatically introduce themselves and sit down for the 'chat'. Where they wanted to know everything about you. In that respect I was glad it so far hadn't happened. Getting information out of me was like trying to get blood from a stone.

Bonnie was assigned to take care of me and so I
followed her into the kitchen where she was handed
back her position of kitchen manager by a lad who was
'acting up' (a term frequently used at Brenten) in her
absences. He wasn't really a candidate for Mr Universe
and clothes show model of the year was definitely out of
the question. He'd got ginger 'out of control' hair,
glasses and ears which were so incredibly large it was
hard to focus on any thing else. To describe his voice
as being upper class would not be giving him full credit.
It was way above me, in fact I thought he could possibly
be foreign! His name, very fittingly, was Nicolas or Nic
to the rest of the crew. I used to work in MacDonalds
during the evening while I was doing school and there
you would be classed as a 'crew member' it reminded
me of the attitude in this kitchen. Full of people trying to
be American. I later found this to be a common
occurrence at Brenten house where words such as 'rap'
and 'fantasy' which I place high on my 'I'd really like to
live in America' list were in very frequent use.

Bonnie thought it would be interesting for me to see how
the kitchen was run. I wish I'd shared the same
enthusiasm. So she had me perch on a stool in the
corner out of the way. Everywhere I went it would
always be me who'd land up with the broken seat and
this was no exception. The last thing I wanted on my
first day was to end up face down on the floor. To avoid
this action I had to keep unnaturally still with one leg at
right angle to the other, balancing the stool on its three
good legs. Such acrobatic talent wasted on a mere
seat.

The other members were briefly introduced and then
work continued as normal I assumed. It was near to tea
time and I was famished until Anth (one of the crew)
rescued something from the oven. The menu described

this as pizza. The hunger pains vanished and in their place came the uneasy feeling of nausea. My appetite had been lost in the rubbish bin, along with the parts of pizza which were beyond repair.

Bonnie was screaming instructions at everybody ordering things to be completed by yesterday. Did it really matter if tea was 5 minutes late I asked (directing the question to anyone who had time to listen)? "Yes" was the answer bluntly contributed in harmony by all occupants of the room. Oh shit why did I have to be so inquisitive. I felt a lecture brewing strongly within Bonnie's lips. Me and my big mouth. I was wrong. Nothing more was said until Nic announced that dinner was served. A surge of people came through the door, pushing and grabbing for the biggest and best things. It was like feeding time on a farm. The dining area was filled with continual chatter largely contributing to the drone which seemed to bounce of the walls each direction meeting in between my ears. Food wasn't on my mind....home was.

I'd left The town where I lived 8 hours previously and already the thought of not being able to see my friends was eating away at my will power. The other residents appeared completely oblivious to what exactly they were eating and when 'seconds' was called the surge reappeared by the 'troughs'. I sat next to Sue who strongly advised me to try some Crème de la Tropic (yogurt and fruit). The kitchen's speciality. When I declined the offer I was ordered to go and fill my bowl and swap it for her empty one. Apparently this delicacy was more sought after than gold dust. I myself could not see the attraction.

I'll never forget the first night I spent at Brenten House. After tea was 'community TD 'and 'showers'. I still don't know what the 'TD' stands for but whenever it was mention everybody hurried along to their assigned positions and cleaned the area from top to bottom. Standards had to be 100% at all costs. I was told to stay put in the lounge for an 'assessment rap chat'. I looked around the room in which six or seven other people were. This included the bloke who had arrived at the same time as me. It was at this point I had my first sighting of a member of staff. We were ordered to make a circle with our chairs. The whole process was done very quietly. We sat and waited, and then….she spoke. Her name was Kristen (I'd gathered this only because each time I asked if there was any staff at all the reply was always "well Kristen's here". It was unlikely that she could have been a resident. She'd got grey hair. Saying that I did notice one or two silvery tones on Sue's head which certainly weren't highlights. Is that what heroin did to a thirty year old?

My first impression of Kristen was she obviously enjoyed these little 'power drive' sessions. It was where she could flash off all her expensive rings and necklaces knowing damned well we'd had our jewellery taken away. She sat and smoked tailor made cigarettes while I struggled relentlessly with trying to conjure up something which vaguely resembled a roll up rather than the trumpets I had been managing. For the next hour I acted as an observer. Kristen could say pretty much what she wanted to anyone of us. All we could do was agree. One lad questioned her comment which proved a mistake. He received a boring and lengthy seminar on the attitude towards Brenten and his high opinion of himself. I was only to pleased to keep quiet. If Kristen had begun to treat me like shit I would probably have replied in the same far from complimentary tone and produced more. Still everything which happened at Brenten was strange. It all seemed over strict.

The rest of the evening also followed a set plan. I had absolutely no time to myself. I think this was the general idea as when found alone you were accused of 'spacing out'. The Americanisms of the place was gradually pissing me off now. Towards the end of the evening my leg which had been twitching all day got worse. I started to feel out of breath. I wasn't in hospital now. I wasn't entitled to feel poorly. Bonnie asked me if I was ok. I couldn't lie about how I was feeling anymore and so desperately replied "NO". she suggest we leave the room which I was only too happy to oblige to. I knew I was having a panic attack but this didn't make it any easier for me to cope with. When I was in hospital I felt safe. If it got to hard to handle there was always the valium to fall back on which in a way was a lovely treat. They gave me such a lift I could escape for a while.

It's understandable how people become reliant upon them. Now there was nothing, no pills, no nurse, and no one who knew how to help me through it. I no longer felt safe but scared and very lonely. This made me worst. Sitting in the dining area I could feel my hands slowly going numb. I found it strange each time this happened. My fingers would stiffen and fix in a position. I was unable to break. The action wasn't unexpected but very uncomfortable. Both Bonnie and Sue tried to help but when someone says" don't worry there's nothing to be afraid of here" it really doesn't ease the feeling. I was grateful for the concern. It would have been worse if I was alone. My face began its sequence of twitches and jerks with the numbness hitting my lips and tongue and cheeks. Before I never felt this bad. Anxiety was a bastard feeling.

Sue thought it would be a good idea for me to lie on the floor. I thought not but agree with her as argument at this stage was to much effort. It was at the moment Kristen entered. You could almost smell the air of authority around her. Earlier in the evening I had been allowed my one phone call for the month. I'd phoned the hospital to let them know I had arrived. It had been nice to here the voice of some I knew. Kristen seeing that I was in a slightly distressed state suggested it would be nice for me to ring there everyday for a while just until I settled in a bit. I wasn't one for accepting special favours but here I was willing to make the exception to every rule. It shocked me to see someone like Kristen with such a mouth on her saying something nice. I appreciated the gesture. Although each phone call made was listened to by a 'senior' resident the thought of still being able to communicate with the outside world was the most comforting I'd heard since I arrived that afternoon. Soon after Kristen's contribution the numbness drifted away leaving me tired and truly embarrassed. For the day to end there would have been a relief. Unfortunately there was still our daily diary to complete.

Questions came thick and fast when I re entered the lounge. Sue handled the over inquisitive lads stating only that I'd been 'dealing with my feelings'. What more could be said? When bed time was eventually called it rang through my ears like sweet music. I crawled into bed and snuggled up to the security of my duvet. Although tired to the extreme I laid awake for hours, over and over again thinking of the day's antics. I felt as if I'd been at Brenten a lifetime. Thinking of my old friends. When I closed my eyes it was easier to image me back there. It's where I wanted to be. In between sleep I repeatedly asked the question was the extent of strictness here real or could I just be in a rather lengthy nightmare. I know which I hoped it was.

Once I realised that the continual poking on my back was not a part of the dream I was having I thought I'd better open my eyes to inquire the origin of this annoying action. After three pathetic attempts my eye was slowly raised. I always wondered if it was possible to get cranes fitted to your eyebrows, that way waking up would be much less effort. My first sighting was of Sue who certainly didn't look her best in the morning. I wasn't sure what the time was. We had no clocks. In a distraught slur I questioned Bonnie. It felt as if I'd just gone to sleep. "6:45" she replied. Jesus, I had only just gone to bed. It was still the middle of the night to me. Was this a practical joke they played on all new residents? "Get out of bed, we'll be late". The tone in Sue's voice was extremely persuasive. I rolled over and slumped on to the floor. Late for what, what was she talking about? It really was too early for all this secrecy. "Can I have a bath?" I was amazed at how polite I sounded; usually if I was disturbed in the middle of my sleep the only words available in my vocabulary were either rude or obnoxious. "NO"...the first contribution from Bonnie. This place got worse. If I didn't bath or shower in the morning I didn't wake up. It was as simple as that.

While I was getting dressed Sue was busy dusting the room and making her bed. Bonnie had already disappeared downstairs. As kitchen manager she had the added responsibliltiy of breakfast...on time. For the next fifteen minutes I tried with no success to get all the creases out of my sheets. Every speck of dust had to be removed. Sue took over my bed making stressing that if standards were not 100% the room would be picked out and us put on a 'bum squad'. She had hoovered and dusted in places I didn't even know existed let alone got dirty.

We managed to get downstairs just before 7:30am so had time for a quick smoke. It was here I received the explanation of what a 'squad' meant. When I had first arrived at Brenten there were two chaps with painting overalls on working outside. I assumed they was builders and didn't think any more of it. It was only now made clear to me that the two blokes were in fact on 'squads' which consisted of working solidly being watched and questioned without a break. Other residents were obliged to say "excuse me" every time you were near whoever was in overalls. But these were the only words allowed to be spoken. Humiliation played a major part in the programme at Brenten House.

From my first roll-up of the morning I got the most amazing head rush. For those treasured few seconds I felt good. May be rollies weren't such a bad idea.

My first complete day at Brenten was spent with my 'peers' (that was everyone else in the assessment session). It was a relief in the respect that they mostly shared the same opinion of Brenten as me. I spent a lot of time talking to Neil. He was the chap who'd arrived the same day as me. He'd been sent by the courts like the majority of residents there. It was instead of finishing his sentence for armed robbery and other minor offences. Neil was ok. He'd smuggled cannabis in to the house despite the extent of the search. I didn't see any harm in that. Not compared with the acid and cocaine which had been his habit. We talked about our separate origins and how we felt about the place. I was missing The town where I lived more and more. Neil described Brenten as being worse than a prison, and he knew. Together we couldn't find a good word to say.

Robin was my assessment leader for the day. God what a prat. Pathetic was an understatement. He acted more like a ten year old. This could have been to do with his size. Standing in front of me was a typical tots to teens shopper. His grey hair poked through under the rim of his 'let's pretend I've got a tweed hat' fake. The silver coloured glasses set off his rather ugly features. This bloke thought he was something special, but he wasn't.

Every where I went Robin had to know about it. Even if it was to the toilet. It was so he could account for all the people he was watching when he was asked. This happened after Role Call was called, usually taking place in the lounge. The word meant silence. No smoking and to appear within sight of who ever called it. The response to the command was a loud shout of 'yes' in unison. The line that followed would be "can I have a department check from co-ord". the co-ordinator leader type person would then say "co-ord here" and explain where the people were who hadn't shown. Following this the other group leaders would reply and so forth. It was all very boring process which became annoying after it happened the usual 12 or 13 times a day. It was to make sure nobody had run away.

My only pleasure of the day was playing pool. I was nominated champion much to the dislike of Fender. He was a cockney and it showed. A typical chauvinist. Fender 'hurricane Higgins' (or so he thought) assumed women couldn't play.

It was a regular procedure at Brenten to constantly 'check out feelings' with people. The person involved would say exactly how they felt and you'd simply reply "OK". I had never used this term as I found it a bit stupid, up until the moment I beat Fender. The temptation was too strong. I called Fender over and in a tone with sarcasm breaking through I asked "Hey Fender, Check out feelings?" He replied quickly and confidently "Fuck Off!" It wasn't really the answer I was searching for. Later he returned the question and I was waiting. "Fender darlin, I'm feeling good, really good". There's nothing I enjoy more than a satisfying session of belittling someone.

I was wary of eating the food at Brenten after the episode of pizza on my first day but to my surprise it was nice. You got a good portion and although sometimes it was hard to decipher exactly what you were eating the tastes was guaranteed to be acceptable. Bonnie did a good job in the kitchen teaching her crew how to cook. This was, I expect, more difficult than perhaps people think. You would understand if you saw her workers! The three times food was prepared were the highlight of the day. Time to sit down and relax as best you could. If nothing else. From working all day you worked up a huge appetite and of course being the sort of person I am having to put tucks in all my size 8 clothes I only required small portions or so I tried to kid myself!

There is nothing I like better on a Friday night to snuggle up to a cushion with some tins and watch telly. At Brenten television was the last thing you had a opportunity to watch. I can understand the decline of the booze but no telly on a Friday night? In fact no telly at all, apart from 'Top of the pops' on a Thursday for ½ hour. And the occasional video. Did these people ever enjoy themselves?....."At Brenten you're not here to enjoy, you're here to work on your feelings". Couldn't I have 5 minutes to myself? I would have found it so easy to turn to Sue who had inconviently appeared next to me and say 'piss off' but I truly felt sorry for her. It was plain to see she was trying her utmost to make me feel better and more settled. It wasn't working.

I still hadn't got used to the fact everyone kept hugging each other. Often blokes would sit on the same chair with their arms around each other. I thought it was nice but because it rarely happens in day to day life it was hard to accept. To start with I thought a couple were gay. It wouldn't have bothered me in fact probably the opposite. In The town where I lived a fair number of my friends were gay. I preferred spending time with them rather than my straight friends. My girlfriends were with their respective girl partners and blokes the same. Everyone knew me and left me well alone. At the time drink filled up to much of my time to ever think about having a boyfriend so I was content to be single.

I wasn't used to being hugged so found it very awkward and uncomfortable when Sue launched a bear clinch on me. In hospital I'd had the same trouble. Always shying away if I detected a hug coming my way. It wasn't that I didn't want some one reassuring me but it had never happened before. Now I am afraid to receive any. I suppose I am scared of getting used to it. In case I become dependant on other people. The day might come there wont be anyone available.

The evening was filled in with Mic's life story. He was trying to get off assessment and on to stage one. A requirement for this was to tell the whole house your life story filling the half an hour allocated. I could see if I stayed I would be on assessment for all 18 months. I had trouble reading out my list in a fish and chip shop and that would be in front of maybe 5 people at the most. When it came to public speaking I was always last in line to complete. Toby Wallace was the only black guy there aside from Anth who was mixed race. He was on contract. There were all different types like 'working' 'silence' 'town crier'. His happened to be a 5 minute contract morning and evening where he'd called the house together and express his thoughts. How he was feeling and what he'd made. I'd listened to him 3 times and already it was obvious he became repetitive of his views. Another evening joy I had to withstand.

Time passed inevitably slowly. When diaries were handed out I knew I would be able to rejoin the only place I liked being at Brenten. In bed asleep. There I faced no pressure or questions. After talking to Sue for a bit I finally managed to undress and desperately crawl into my barricade. There I closed my eyes hoping I'd dream good dreams.

Everyone apart from me had been really excited about Saturday coming. There was a change in the usual work program. In the afternoon a fund raising event had been organised to do with a telethon for a national charity. All the morning was spent preparing for this. Dusting, hoovering and general cleaning around the house which wasn't even to be open to the public. The grounds, which were a fair size, also had to be prepared. Robin made a coconut shy which looked more like an attempt at Lego construction. I got lumbered with sweeping up all kinds of shit off the path. This was while Neil dug it out of the gaps between the paving. My finger nails which I'd been growing were now looking rather unattractive and broken. I felt like one of those road sweepers who walked around The town where I lived all day with a broom and cart. The only difference was those trampy blokes did it by choice. Lunch was just a snack as there was not much time due to the preparation of the sausages for hot dogs to sell the visitors. For the afternoon all residents were given two pounds spending money apart from Neil and me who hadn't been there long enough to have anything. It was the first sighting of money for everyone since they'd been at Brenten. It caused a lot of chatter and enthusiasm. It was like an infant's first trip to the sweet shop left to count their pennies. It made me angry and frustrated to see grown up adults act like kids. Most of all I couldn't join in because I didn't have any.

The sea cadets arrived early to set up all their equipment for the band display. Looking around them I wonder which would be the person who hit a wrong note or played in the wrong key. I loved it when that sort of thing happened. I've always found other peoples misfortunes really humorous.

From that moment on I felt small. As more visitors came I shrunk even more. I was contemplating making a stick saying 'I'm an alcoholic not a junkie' as we were made to mingle with the guests. This was so they could see what kind of people came to Brenten. You could tell by the look in people's eyes that they assumed all residents would be heroin addicts. Some people are so blind to their fears. I was cross at being a show piece on display. I felt humiliated and embarrassed. Was I as bad as a junkie? Since I'd been at Brenten I'd felt inferior to the rest. I was the only one, apart from Jack who was there for drinking. Jack had come because when he drank he became violent. He didn't crave so I couldn't understand why he didn't leave it alone. Everyone else had been a user. It made me feel as if I'd not really got a problem and that I shouldn't need help. Sometimes I wondered if I had a fix whether that would make me one of the crowd. It was then I first seriously considered leaving Brenten. I hadn't got anywhere to go but there was no way I was staying at a place which to me projected the need of taking hard drugs.

The rest of the day I spent totally oblivious to what was going on around me. Instead I went over the possibilities of a place I could stay if I left. Tuesday would be a good day to leave. My rail ticket was valid for the middle 3 days of each week. Could I wait that long? My thoughts were broken into by a blast from the makeshift disco unit. The guy DJ ing was trying to be Bruno Brooks which I would have thought wasn't much of an ambition. The fellas had organized a log race where they all dressed up looking total pricks and carried logs across a course. To me the afternoon was a flop. There wasn't many people show up and those who did were all the sort from rich up-bringing. It was humiliating and an experience I won't be keen to undergo again.

That evening we had the added excitement of a horror video. I declined the offer of blood and guts and retreated into the annex where Fender 'cocky' decided to degrade me even more. I was wound up anyway and the last thing I needed was some bastard who thought his excessive amount of grease in his hair made him over attractive, telling me how I felt. How should he bloody know? He knew absolutely nothing about me yet insisted on airing his views. Who gave him the right to judge me? After a matter of days, weeks, months... I sure as hell didn't know but wasn't prepared to listen to a load of shit coming from an ex-user.

My worst objection was that along side feeling inferior I also felt that I was better than the others. I hadn't lowered myself to the extent of needing to inject. Deep down I knew I was just as bad. Only I had depended on other stuff. At least drinking was legal when you were over 18. Even so I had been drinking more and more since I was 13 and still I was not of age. I went over and over it in my mind. Who was I trying to convince and prove something to. Me or them?

We were allowed to go to bed later on a Saturday but I was so knackered I didn't care. Milky coffee was brought up to our rooms as a thank you for the day. It was the first time I'd had coffee and the welcome taste lingered for ages. Bonnie unsure of whether to trust me or not, expressed the need for a cigarette. There was no smoking in the dormitories but rules had never stopped me before. Mind the penalty was a little steeper to what I was used to. I was only to glad to participate though. At least this showed a sign of some human activity. After blocking all possible escape routes for the smoke we sat and puffed deviously. It was how I imagined life at a boarding school to be. The crafty fag. A minor difference was that Bonnie was 37.

So I had managed to complete another day at Brenten and then another and so it went on. My fantasy of leaving was now developing quickly to reality as the hours, days, weeks slipped by. Tuesday was coming, which Tuesday I didn't know but it felt like the great escape. We had a lay in Sunday mornings until 8:00am...it was a welcome gesture though. Still too early for my liking. The rest of the day was boring and mundane. Much the same as every other. What kept me going during that morning was the thought of roast pork for lunch. I loved food, especially roast potatoes. This made the letter group almost bearable. This group was held on Sundays and Wednesday's. You had an hour in which time incoming letters were read out in front of your 'peers' and the same for letters waiting to be sent. Toby Wallace was our group leader. He assumed his authority gave him the right to mock all our group. I didn't like Toby much. He was acting so big until the times of his contract then he had to stand up and really make a prick of himself. I enjoyed that bit. Toby really needed taking down a peg or two. I'd been building my hopes up continuously thinking there was a chance I might get a letter. There was four letters and three of us waiting. One of them had to be for me. Toby handed them out. Where was mine? I had a sick feeling inside of me. Nothing, no bloody letter. Had they confiscated it?....i wasn't sure cos they could. The disappointment it left me with is inexplicable. I felt more alone than ever. This was the last straw enhancing my determination to leave one day. I sat oblivious to the voices reading out their individual letters. Toby searched the envelopes giving off the impression he was almost wanting to find something he could take away. The end of the session was near leaving me with barely enough time to read the letter I had prepared. As I read only the bits I wished to out loud I knew it would be read again. Would they appreciate my descriptions of sarcastic hellos? Probably not, nobody seemed to have an ounce of humour at Brenten.

Ivon entered the room announcing the end of the group. He was about the best looking guy. Another dwarf, he was part of the co-ord team and made sure everybody knew that and treated him accordingly. His looks were the only thing he had going for him. His personality stank! Though very boring the session had gone too quickly for my liking, not leaving enough time for the second letter I was hoping to send. There were no favours at Brenten. It would just have to wait until the next letter group.
Roast pork dinner was like having all my Christmases come at once. With a second helping thrown in it made Brenten seem almost humane. The sense of being in

paradise soon ended and in its place returned frustration anger and fear. I wanted to be free of this place. Sometimes I thought about staying...like there was a choice rather than being forced to be here. 18 months wasn't such a long time. Not compared to the rest of my life. That's what everyone at Brenten kept telling me. Most of the residents had been through years of party rebellion and everything else which accompanies the pleasures of growing up. I hadn't! for Christ sake I was going to miss out on the rest of my teens if I stayed forever. With that came the thought that my official adult birthday of 18 would be spent sweeping floors or such like. Why couldn't every one accept the fact I was still a kid.

I wasn't any worse off (probly far better off) than the other residents all having their individual problems but I felt it. I was content to sit and wallow in my own self pity until the day I escaped. Nothing anybody said to me made any sense. I was totally disinterested in working on my 'feelings'. The only way I knew how to snap out of a mood such as this was to go and get plastered. Which was exactly what I was going to do as soon as I was free.

The Sunday afternoon was spent in the kitchen. The assessment team was volunteered as everyone else was due to participate in a 'group'. One had taken place earlier that week and from what I could gather they were pretty hairy. We were under close observation from Jones and Drayten. It wasn't too bad. Jones and Drayten both lived in the cottage. It was known as pre re-entry. I was so jealous of them. It was easy for Drayten to say "stick at the program, it's worth it in the end". He'd already been through 9 months of sheer hell. After that he had 2 months of almost bearable living. It could only get better and with the excitement of moving into the Terrace, the re-entry stage of the program in the not too distant future. His views would obviously be optimistic. Drayten and Jones had every right to be conceited about their achievements. It made it no less difficult to accept though.

By the end of that afternoon I was feeling pretty bored with their repetitive statements of encouragement. Their air of authority became almost choking. Did they have any faults? Envy ate away at any trace of determination I had left in me.

One evening was spent listening to the relaxing music of Toby 'I'm better than a pop star' Wallace and his guitar. The closest collective term describing the music Toby was playing would I think be 'blues'. His instrumental skills were impressive. His vocal ability was not. Each new song he attempted was familiar as an up tempo version of his previous rendition. Singing about lost love and all his hurt and suffering. You could really see Brenten had made him optimistic to the extreme! I was miserable and bored. Applause and requests for an encore faded away. Fresh fruit was bought round and diaries were handed out. I traded my apple for a rolli off Sue. I didn't like to mention it but her fingers seemed enlarged daily. I'm glad my fingers don't look like over generously sized chipolatas.

One Monday morning Bonnie was promoted to act as part of the co-ord team replacing Ivon who had been knocked of his perch at the top. He was now a gardens crew, not a manager or assistant, just a crew member. His gnome like features may have aided the decision! Humiliation was written all over Ivon's face. His authority had been stolen. It caused a few angry words to the hierarchy which was strictly not allowed. I felt no sympathy for Ivon but like a lot of the other residents great satisfaction at the fact that somebody so head strong could be belittled so quickly. More than likely the general idea of the whole operation at Brenten House.

With the possibility that I would escape occupying my thoughts the last thing on my mind that Monday morning was watering Brenten's home grown attempts at lettuce, cabbage and Rhubarb. Robin insisted we did this daily. Neil and I decided it would be more fun playing 'lets see how wet we can get Robin's trousers before he notices'. It was much more challenging. The weather being slightly less than what was expected in May made it difficult for his trousers to dry quickly. My eye for the target of his knees (an average persons ankle height) had veered away slightly and due to the unfortunately large size of the wet patch I had created Robin for the rest of the morning was thought to be incontinent.

Neil and I got on really well. Both hating the place as much as one another. Being sent by the courts made for less of an option. I told no one I was planning to leave. Not even Neil, although it made me feel guilty leaving him. I decided it was best to keep quiet and continued to water the unattractive cactus, another of Brenten House inspirations.

I opted for a vegetarian lunch dish sometimes as it was a trendy thing to do. I could tell that it was something with eggs in it this one time. That was the extent of the description. The rest was left to my imagination. For what was left of my day things sometimes felt positive. I think because I planning to run and so had less time to tolerate the daily procedures. In the evening we had another assessment rap. If anything I felt extremely smug and content that only I knew my plans for the following days...the account of my 'feelings' in diary time contained no inclination of this I made sure. In bed

I laid patiently waiting to fall into the unconscious state of sleep. I seemed to be awake for hours. Longing for the pint of lager I was to award myself. I think I had decided….tomorrow was the day I was leaving.

"Wake up its 6:50am" The day had arrived. Usually it was a problem for me getting out of bed. That morning it was automatic. Excitement rushed through the length of my body. My adrenalin was high. The great escape was about to commence. I was so confident about my plans I felt the suggestion of rebelling slightly knocking continually at the back of my mind. To hell with making my bed properly. Who cared if there was dust on the bloody pillow? I certainly didn't. Being put on a 'squad' meant nothing today or anymore. I was off and nobody was going to stop me. So leaving my sheets ruffled and my quilt noticeably crooked I left the dormitory. I didn't realise at the time I would not be returning there under any circumstances. As I gloated my way through morning course. The name I had given to each days introduction. Like a school assembly but longer, stricter and so much more boring. I felt satisfied I was about to make the right decision. " you will be on tea duty". My thoughts were broken in to. That's what you think I muttered, biting my cheek so as the massive grin of contentment did not spring on my face and give the game away. Nobody was ever happy doing tea duty. It was like being a waiter for the day in addition to your other tasks.

After every one who had anything to say had finished I announced to Bonnie my request for departure. Her response wasn't as I'd wish. Her voice travelled as if projected through a megaphone. "Clive…She wants to leave!"

Welcome to My World

The residents left in the room stared at me like vultures awaiting attack on their prey. The attention was on me once more. Apart from my first day I hadn't created much of an attraction. That was until now. Jesus I could feel myself bubbling into a crimson mess. I hadn't expected this much interest or resentment. I wasn't sure which.

The constant thought of a refreshing pint dragged me through the situation I had landed myself in but I was unaware of worst still to come. Bonnie took me to the hall way where she passed on my request to Gary. He was leading the in charge team until Bonnie got the hang of things. There was a lot of hush hush conversation where I became extremely paranoid and with every justification. I could hear my name mentioned on numerous occasions. This was without the assistance of my hearing aid! The white bench was brought out and placed directly behind where I was standing. Personally I hadn't used the bench. It signified the thought of leaving if somebody sat on it. Mark was on the bench nearly every day I'd been there so I gathered not many other residents had the opportunity to use it either. The hall was filled with silence for a while. Gary had gone into the staff room. Officially nobody was allowed to talk to me but Bonnie, being the daring type proceeded to say how much she'd like to keep my deodorant and that she hoped I got on all right. Trevor expressed that within two months of leaving Brenten I would be back on the bottle. He was being over generous, I knew I'd be tasting the familiar friendliness of alcohol within two hours…at the most!

Gary reappeared from behind the door leading into the staffs own little palace. In large unattractive letters was the word 'private' centring the tatty lose fitting door. That was the way they like it to stay. He ordered one of the admin crew to summon Sue. She was now gardens manager and very much enjoying the authority. Within minutes she had arrived. She was directed up the stairs to pack my belongings. With a look of horror centred on me she obliged and made her way up the stairs. When I had first arrived at Brenten, Sue had pointed out the fact I walked with a limp and that she had a bad leg. One evening when we were both in bed the subject arose again. Sue explained that one day when she had run out of arm, wrist and neck veins to inject in to, a friend suggested the top of her leg. The person who injected her missed the vein and caught an artery. This left Sue with some poorly long word thing and a request from the hospital to amputate her left leg. She refused but is now left with big chunks taken out and considerable pain. As Sue walked up the stairs with her bum screaming to be let out of the under amply sized jeans the stretched material emphasised her injury and showed off the seriousness of the damage. It was a pretty ugly sight. Gary looked at me in sheer disgust and suggested I sit on the bench. I declined the offer expressing my decision to leave was not just a 'feeling'. I did not feel it necessary to be put through any further humiliation by being seated on the bench. The reply came from Bonnie and was backed up by Gary. "if you don't sit on the bench you leave Brenten with out any of your possessions" satisfaction biting with each word. I wasn't going to stand for any more bullshit from these 'nothingness' people and stated that withholding my possessions was in fact stealing and if this idea was carried out would certainly become a police matter. I surprised myself with the extent of big words I had thrown in to make it sound good. Really I hadn't a bloody clue what it meant.

Throughout the waiting game for my possessions Bonnie tried to retain some kind of authority over me.

She said I wasn't to lean against the wall. Immediately I carried out the opposite. She told me not to smoke...so I smoked. I just couldn't believe the cheek of the woman. I had no reason to follow orders especially from an ex junkie!

Soon after my small confrontation with Bonnie my clothes arrived. Untidily thrown into cheap bin liners. I began to search through making sure everything had been collected. Soon I realised a number of clothes were missing. Was it worth the trouble of another argument? I couldn't see the need. They were only material things and could be replaced, I was too interested in getting out of the prison camp. Sue waltzed past me wearing a blue t-shirt which was also missing that was one thing accounted for. Bonnie mentioned that I was going to be taken to Sharfield station by Zeta, one of the staff. She was Dutch or something. I'd seen her once but never spoke with her. She was big and blonde. Not unlike a lot of Dutch women! I had to wait until she was ready which Gary said would be another hour.

To everyone who walked past me during the following hour I was no longer someone trying to make a fresh start unaided by drugs. By now I had become a total failure, a minute dreg in the used teabag people called society. They were making a bloody good job of making me feel guilty and a let down. Suddenly all the promises I'd made to my friends before I left came flooding back. Swamping me and leaving me unsure once again of the decision I had made. It was realistically too late to turn back and I didn't want to but so many questions posed openly in my mind. Had I tried my hardest? Did I give the project a chance? I'd messed up badly now. If I returned to Home I would have to explain. No one would believe the extent of strictness here. How would I explain the reasons for 'giving up'? That's what I'd done. Given up on for the first time in my life apart from the odd game of eye spy. How could I handle this amount of failure. The only way I knew was to drink. The craving began. One drink wouldn't hurt? Maybe even get sloshed. Just the once. I'd realised I had a problem, surely I could handle it now? No problem!.

Before long Mark appeared off his squad. Removing the bench from behind me and placing it down opposite. It was obviously that time of the day. Some one was ordered to pack Mark's belongings which I think shocked him slightly. His mind had been made up for him. Through sign language we arranged to meet in the nearest pub to Sharfield train station at 1pm. It never came off. I was unaware whether Mark actually left or not. This Tuesday happened to be an open day at Brenten for professional judges so reluctantly I was ushered into a corner. I couldn't be bothered to make a spectacle of myself although it did enter my mind for a while. That last hour I spent at Brenten House was only bearable due to the fact I had made the desire to drink again.

Zeta instructed me to her rather flash fiesta sport where I sat feeling small, ashamed and nervous. Apart from going for a drink I hadn't planned my next move. I'd got money which was essential. It would be a waste not to view more of the southern area. Portland, Portsmouth…something with a port sounded the best bet. Yes that was my next destination. Where in Portland? As Zeta pulled away I remember that every breath I took pierced the silence which crowded the car.

I surprised myself when the words started escaping from my lips. "Thanks for giving me the chance!" Why was I trying to justify myself?

"It's just a shame" Zeta responded.
"Were you a junkie" I asked, not sure what to expect. The next 5 minutes were heart breaking. Zeta explained she had been an alcoholic since she was 17. She had been national sports champion of Holland in martial arts. I explained I also had done bits for 7 years to a high standard. We had so much in common.

"Yes" she replied "apart from the fact I've done something about it."

I felt I'd been reduced to nothing. How degrading. If only I had known before that I wasn't alone at the rehab centre.
"At Brenten you learn to ask!"
I was gob smacked...why couldn't I have found out. She drew up at the station. As I opened the door I expressed my regret for leaving and I was grateful for the chance.
"Take care of yourself; I hope you will be ok"
The car pulled away and I was left alone. The tears began to roll frantically down my cheeks. I'd messed up again only this time it was all my doing. I'm not sure whether I missed Brenten despite all the torture. At least it was somewhere. But now I was left without anything once more....where was the pub?

Chapter Seven

I looked up at comedy girl. She sat not really waiting for me to say anything, she just sat. "Weren't you the jumped up teenager trapped in some lesbian dungarees just screaming to get out?" I said it with sarcasm ribbing through. My face smiling.
"You think?" she replied equally as sarcastically. "That's why I didn't want to tell you that bit. I wanted you to read it as I saw it happening. What's scary is I paid such little attention to the running of the unit. The rules were like nothing I have ever experienced then or since. The patronising ways.

The philosophy was to reduce the person to nothing. That's why they took jewellery, personal effects, anything that made up part of you they took. Theory was they would then rebuild you minus what ever vice you had been sent there for. I was scared. Some of the bits I still remember now I have not mentioned in that story which I find weird. The way you were made to act out some obscure character and sing and dance in front of the whole group. To make you feel silly and stuff. They were some of the punishments for breaking the rules. And that squad thing. I have so understated that. It was literally from the minute you woke like 6.30. you got a few minutes for breakfast, lunch and tea and that was it. You were outside in the grounds in your orange overalls doing, well whatever had been chosen for you to do. "

"What like?" I queried.

"Anything really from cutting the acres of grass with nail scissors to picking up the leaves from the large amount of trees with a pair of tweezers. You name it, all to make you feel small...but I just fought them the whole way. Crazy thing is all of the people who were on the programme had as I said been sent to finish off their sentences from prison. All bar one had directly or indirectly been responsible for somebody else dying, well that's what I'd gathered from listening"

My face requested the explanation, I didn't need to ask for it in words…
"I mean some people had driven cars when they were high and crashed in to people and they had been killed. Some had killed their friends through similar driving accidents. A couple had injected mates and miss hit. A couple had O.D. ed their friends by accident. Some had committed robbery and this had gone wrong and people had been killed. They'd seen mates die with the needle still sticking out of the eye ball. It was hard core, well I thought it was. The place was full to overflowing which meant 41 or 42 people all with there own horrible story, all wanting to find a better way. Some wanting to return to prison cos…it was better. I hated the place and everything that it was about.

I wrote more to that story but I haven't shown you. Probably because its difficult to make sense of what I'm saying. Think maybe I was so stoned when I wrote it I was only worried about the décor on the walls of the hotel. Stuff like that and to be fair, what happened after I left the rehab centre for a while was just a little bit too wild."

"You seem so different now. Not so….angry I suppose" I wanted comedy girl to talk some more about it but I sensed I'd had my lot where the rehab adventure was concerned.

"Yes I am different now. I was full of life and I really believed I was right and the rest of the world was just stepping stones to where I wanted to get to. I believed that every thing was simple and honest. I suppose I believed in the fairy tale. Stuff leading up to the rehab centre and that little episode they were all just chapters, all stuff that was kind of ok in the messed up world of growing up. The stuff that happened when I came home, that wasn't quite so gorgeous"

I shifted my numb cheek over slightly on my bar stool throne. I sensed some more of chunky oh not so chunky's life lessons were coming up. More coffee was ordered. I wasn't going anywhere fast and my coffee companion was getting ready to tell some more.

"So I returned, well I returned to the hospital, was quickly moved on, which suited me fine, to a strange but convenient set up. It was a family home quite large. I had my own room and a kettle. There was a jar of coffee mixed with chicory as a present left in there. I'd never heard of chicory so I thought that was proper posh. The lady, never knew her name, was trying to be nice to me but I wouldn't really let her. She offered to cook my tea and do my washing. I didn't want any help with that stuff. I didn't last long there as it felt a bit false. Think maybe I made it that way. Got a job not a great one but it was full time and I could do it.

Moved back to the hostel where I lived before and stuff was just getting back to normal. I wasn't drinking anymore and I was doing ok. The hostel was like 'growing up' school. Before the detox thing and after we just had a riot. The combination of people who lived there made for so many crazy times. Good ones and some, I suppose, not so good but they all seemed to make up parts of our day. Kirsty was 16 too. She came to stay not long after to me. She would hang out with some boys from the other side of town. I liked Kirsty, she was fun. She got a job as a chef and went off to travel with the company. I thought that was brilliant. A few weeks before she left on her adventure she'd walked in to a bit of trouble. It wasn't just a bit at all really. I think it was huge but then like I say it made up part of one day."

"What was it?" I asked, curious to have some understanding of the hostel life, (although I was getting the picture).

"Well I was hanging around, playing a bit of pool and stuff. It was late but then that's when the hostel was truly alive. Kirsty walked in, a bit sluggish I suppose but no different from any of us determined to put one foot in front of the other loaded with booze. She'd been over the other side of the town with the lads she knew. She joined me at the pool table. Bit pale, bit wobbly, bit normal really. When I started to speak to her it wasn't so gorgeous. I said ' alright kirst?' and she, cool as a cucumber replied ' well yeah but I've been stabbed.' I immediately done 'surprised eyes' (which wasn't helpful) and then said 'have you?' (again not my sharpest action.) Once over the initial 'I have to say crap' stuff, I got her to show me where she was hurting. She had a pretty impressive puncture wound and blood to match. We got her to the hospital and she got sorted. We didn't call the police. We were busy getting pissed.

I knocked around a lot with Shirl. She was a wild one, fantastic. She carried a lot of family baggage. Stuff with her dad and shotgun. Other stuff too, her brother, think he'd hung himself? We used to chat about it, thing was we were so mashed it all became easy to ignore....for then. Anyway Shirl used to knock on my door each morning to get me up for school. She was at college so was getting up anyway. I'd open the door to a bracardi getting friendly with a splash of coke and all busy caressing some ice. Sometimes we'd get a little carried away and only make it as far as downstairs. Sometimes we'd make it to the pub. The new drinking laws had only just arrived. A gift... I did use to pop into school sometimes but that kind of stopped after a little bit of a wild one. Shirl and Dodge, he was one of two others that made up our bar quartet. They thought it would be fab to give me a little hair style. Needless to say apparently I was all for it, no recollection of that, not a scrap. So I wake up to find I have long, bright red, (pillar box I think they called it,) hair. Not only that but underneath the longness they had shaved off all the rest, sides and back. It wasn't the prettiest gift anyone had ever surprised me with. School said I wasn't allowed there til it was sorted. I found myself too busy to sort it for ages.

You see, Shirl used to get a bundle of money each month. It was, well I suppose like a pay off from her mum. It used to go in a pot along with my wages, I worked some nights after school, Dodge put money in the pot and so did Will, he was the fourth member. All we had to do then was drink it!

My work were really kind to me and I was rubbish at it. I think maybe because I was quite often wasted. One day I woke up at about 4am on the floor in the bakery that was the basement of the restaurant café where I served. I think I came straight from a night in town. The creepy baker man who saw no one because of his unsocial hours was really pleased I was there. I never want to explore why that was! The manager was so strict but still used to bag up some of the stuff we ordinarily had to throw out (the rules) for me to take home to eat. I was glad for that. I didn't have a coat and without telling me her and her sidekick took a little bit out of my money each week. Then one day they got me a coat, I was so glad for that. They were kind to me when I should have been sacked probably five times over. I loved working there.

We had a basement at the hostel which we filled with gym stuff. Dodge taught me how to use nunchuks. He was really good at them. He had the proper ones, so no padding on them. They really hurt when you done it wrong. I learnt fast how to use them. Dodge rocked he would teach me all sorts of kung fu stuff. He was so cool.

Gary, another lad would do nunchuks at midnight in the carpark out the front. He would do it bare chested. He, however was not even close to cool. Gary was a bit of a fruit loop. One day he walked into the local hospital with a big old bag and said it was a bomb. He didn't stay at the hostel after that.

Will had to leave because his job took him elsewhere. Shirl went with him. Me and Dodge used to go and see them sometimes, he always looked out for me. It used to be wild. Together we all made so many smiles. But things change you know. I hate change. Shirl somehow ended up in a mental place, like a locked one. Maybe life got too heavy? Dodge died, he killed himself one day. Anyway..."

Comedy girl was leaving no room for me to comment. So I respected that and waited silently for her to continue.

Chapter Eight

"I was doing ok until my birthday that is. It was my 18th"

"I was doing ok until my birthday that is. It was my 18th and so some of the boys thought it would be a great idea if we smoked a bit and got wasted. I of course thought it was a marvellous alternative to my now drink free world. Before the 'detox' thing I used to get stoned often. My room mate Ellie punk rocker had taught me a great deal. We would get smashed. She was much older than me and always going to be fashion designer. She was off the wall and I loved her. We were in our room one evening pretty mashed up when there was a knock at the door. It was the warden, not the beast, it was the old one who actually was in charge. She was always pissed and angry at the world but I liked her loads, she was kind to me, in a cross way, but still kind. She wanted the door open and me and Ellie were half way though a big old reefer. Not quite knowing where to put the evidence I opened the top draw and Ellie threw the joint. It was my tampax box that caught it. The draw remained open and the warden came in. "I can smell something herbal" she stated.

Its jos sticks Miss M both Ellie and I replied in unison. We laughed hard as somehow during our session we had started saying everything with the letter 'k' in front of it. This had continued in our reply to Miss M. She stared, we laughed some more. She turned to the draws and stared. Ellie and I followed her stare. All three of us were now looking at the tampax box smoking away (and smiling just a bit). Me and Ellie laughed some more proper belly laughs. Ellie did a little wee in her pants by accident because she was laughing hard. We laughed at that to. Miss 'M' retreated saying for us to stop burning the jos sticks now. Ellie changed her pants and we carried on smoking stuff. It was a riot, the stuff growing up memories are made of.

Welcome to My World

So the whole joint thing should be fun. It all should have been great fun. But it wasn't. A couple of the lads had just come back from doing a 'smash and grab' at a jeweller's in town (oh how I wish this was just to make the story more meaty and not true at all). They were lads I wasn't as close to but they came along for the ride. They rolled my joint. I had a 'special' one because it was birthday eve. And that's where things went tits up. The shit they'd put in it was so very special it sent me tripping like I had never tripped before. They laughed I didn't. Things were different this time it was so harsh and it didn't stop...not forever. They never told anyone what they'd messed it up with. It didn't matter how many times they were asked. Those lads thought it was their secret to keep. It changed my world.

I was pretty proper poorly for ages. Spent days in bed couldn't do a lot. Eventually I dragged my arse to the doctors and got some diazepam. Nothing was very regulated then not like now. It was four or five weeks maybe more, eight or nine weeks shit I don't know but it was some time before anyone realised I shouldn't be taking quite so many for quite so long. As I remember I floated a good 8 or 9 pills a day...they helped I think!!!!"

"So when eventually it was realised that someone had done a bit of a whoopsy in the prescribing department I was invited back to the Looney bin to 'support me' they called it whilst the medicine was sorted. I can remember arriving, I can remember being handed some orange stuff to take, the rest has been filled in by others as that's where my memory runs out. The doctors or whoever, in their infinite wisdom had thought it best to stop all the diazepam immediately. Nice choice I felt.....kinda not. Instead the 'orange' magic was given. I apparently reacted a little badly to that, was told after that the drug hadn't suited me."

Comedy girl looked up from her coffee cup and caught my glance. I could sort of guess what had happed to her, I was almost sure I knew the drug she was referring to. A really old one that's no longer used. She said she didn't want to think anymore about it and I understood why.

She continued "So the days turned into weeks but not many. Drama teacher had returned and clearly taken advantage of my incapacity at points and again I was let out. This time under the care of a new shrink who had arrived from overseas. Outpatient appointments aplenty I entered back into my world. And so I carried on. Got another job and was fairly good at it. Hooked up with a couple of lads and we used to play pool all night at a local café. Now that had some viewing pleasures. It was like 'on the buses' green room. Odd looking people with odd looking lives. Counting the days to their next dole check and just waiting to have the money lifted off them as they lost at the pool table time and time again. From there we'd go straight to work, grab a few hours sleep in the afternoon, and so it continued. I was doing ok. "

The pace had slowed of comedy girls story. Nothing sounded to shocking or horrific. Rather tame compared with her previous antics. A sense of disappointment chased my thoughts. Had she ran out of story....?

"Do you know, I've met some weird and wonderful people? All this chat, it's got me thinking. The hostel was a collecting point for them, just as the café was. How do I manage to find these people? Fantastic. At the hostel there was an older guy. Not like 100 years old but old to me. Probably 45 ish? He used to be a member of the ...."

Comedy girl lent towards me, she got ever so close, wasn't sure if she was going to do a little kiss. I lent towards her, so not wanting the kiss thing to happen. I was safe...it was a whisper! And so she whispered in my ear..
"IRA"

Unfortunately I forgot the whole whisper technique and repeated loudly "IRA".

"Yes" she said, "shhh a bit. He was proper in it. I was a little bit frightened of him but he was a nice man who you did not upset. Instead I would sometimes drink whiskey with him.

There was a boy called Trevor too. He was convinced he was in the army and for months so were we. He used to go off to work every day. He had all the kit. No one had a reason to doubt him. That was until we were walking through town. Me, Trev and Muffin, she was doing something dance like at a college. Anyway as we walked through the town a car made that back-firing noise. So immediately Trev drops to the floor in a strange Rambo type position and pretends to hold a rifle. Muffin and I clearly had to laugh at that...for quite sometime. Trev reckoned it was his army training made him do that. Shortly after the 'Rambo drop down' manoeuvre we found out Trev worked at a petrol station on the American base. He was a cashier. Do you know I could go on for hours with different names, different faces. Everyone had a story behind them...."

I needed to get Comedy girl/Story teller extraordinaire back on track. So I prompted her "So you were saying, everything was going ok. You were doing a bit of pool hustling, working a bit...yeah?"

"Yes sorry, I haven't thought about those people for ages, anyway yes, I attended the appointments to keep the shrink happy and that was that. I had applied for my nurse training and things were really kicking into gear.

Chapter Nine

I don't know when it was when I started to think things were a bit strange where the shrink thing was concerned. After all, the doctor tells you and….consequently you do it. The young one I had met in hospital used to hang out with us sometimes and also had to attend the outpatient thing. We had appointments one after the other and this one time I remember her coming out and stating she had been put on the medication and the dose etc. It wasn't until I came out and realised I had exactly the same medication to take and the same dose. Only our things were heaps different. It made me think for a minute but that was it. The next time I had more medication, lots more. And so this became a pattern. Have to say I felt pretty shit but I was starting to associate the fact that each time I said it wasn't great I got more and more drugs. Not in a good way.

One day at work I felt really crap, physically I was a mess. I can remember my mum helped me get to the doctors. He was a nice man. He was also very surprised by all the medicine I was taking. He took blood from me. He said there was an error and that the medicine was making me poorly. Maybe it had been written wrong. He said my blood was toxic. I didn't know what he meant. All I heard was that he was sending me back to the shrink to make it all alright. I didn't want to go. It always resulted in more medication. It was becoming predictable. I wasn't enjoying this process any but all I knew was the shrink told me if I didn't take the pills I would be made to. There was never anyone else there in the room. Just me and the shrink. She said she could do anything, and I supposed she could.

I was looking forward to my nursing course, I had been accepted and it was in a different town so I would be able to move a way from the Looney house shrink who I didn't like at all. All the pills made me feel weird like horrible stuff and I was so scared not to take them as some how I thought they would know. It got so I couldn't work stuff out easily. Was I getting more poorly? You know proper mental? Inside, deep down I didn't think so. Sometimes I could hear that deep thought. Sometimes all I could here was the Plum Lip Shrink telling me I didn't know shit and that I was wrong.

When I went I always said I was fine and that still resulted in an extra tablet here or there. I can remember them all. The colours, the size, everything."

I listened to comedy girl in horror. It sounded a bit crazy and that she was almost being used as a bit of a drug dummy toy. Some meds can result in awful physical symptoms. It sounded like she wasn't being monitored and of course she would get poorly.

"When did it all stop" I asked her. "Surely some one noticed something? Did you need it all?"

"Well my doctor, you know, GP, had stressed he would let the shrink sort it all out. And because of that he didn't need to see me."

"What was the shrink's name?" I asked, he sounds like a bit strange.

"It was a she. She always wore Plum. I don't want to say her name. I don't want to think about her. She was poison. It kind of all stopped all of a sudden. But not before the worst bit."

Welcome to My World

I was waiting for a punch line from comedy girl. Something to bring back the funnies. Some bizarre story or a patient twist but nothing came. The mood was suddenly different. I asked for more from my companion.

"Look she doesn't need a name. That way I get to keep something secret. You know private to me. If you search long enough you'll find out more but not from me. Her lipstick....that was plum too. It paved the way for some of my scariest nightmares. Her voice full of accent. Her eyes were piercing but when you tried to explore them....they were full up of empty.

Anyway by the time things got really hairy I was as I say looking forward. New job, new home, new everything. I had to go for an appointment with shrink plum lips. Not for any reason, they had become more frequent as had the medicines. I hated it. The route that made up my morning noon and night doses. I hated the sick feel that accompanied them and the rest of the trip it seemed to create. Some days I really thought I was going mad. Seeing things, all sorts of crap was going on. By the time that appointment had come I was up to nearly 30 tablets a day, all of different colour shape and use...supposedly. Some made me thirsty like you couldn't satisfy. Not ever. Some made my dreams so scary I was grateful for the day. Some made my head feel heavy, some made my thoughts cloudy. Unless that was all me?...but it wasn't.

So I went that day after I finished my shift. I was keen to see the back of plum lip shrink. I said as I always did I was doing fine and that maybe I didn't need to come so often. Her reply was ....well confusing at first. She said she thought I needed to come into hospital for a while. That I was really sick and that I needed more medicines. I'd just finished my shift at work, I worked full time. I never had a sick day only the toxic thing. Why was she saying I was sick. My first thought was I am mad. I don't know I'm sick and I'm a fruit loop. I think everything is ok and I can work. That's what happens to mad people. They don't know they are mad. That thought only lasted seconds. I knew I wasn't mad. I knew I was doing ok considering the huge amount of rubbish that was being pumped into me. I said no thanks to her. I was scared of her and a bit trapped in as much as my own doctor wouldn't touch my drugs. He said she was the professional. I tried to make the appointment end saying I would book another one, in? I queried how many weeks. Plum lips spoke in the horrible accented voice I can still hear. You need to be admitted and if you are refusing then you will be sectioned. The woman was crazy. I'd been at work this morning and now suddenly she was suggesting a section. I'd been there remember. I told her no, I told her I was ok, and that it wasn't fair to try and make me stay. She called her bitch. I call him that because he was. In walked a wet nose boy man with black rim glasses and big trousers. He never spoke to me once, he never looked at me. She gave him a piece of paper and said sign it. He did and then left the room.

The next couple of hours were wild but in a bad way. The shrink woman kept me in a room. Unbeknown to me at the time my mum had been phoned…anonymously. How very Sherlock Holmes I thought."

At last a breath of comedy girl had returned. It seemed like forever since she had lightened the air with wit. She continued.

"My mum had phoned my sister and when I reached the ward full of objections they were already there. They were confused too. Plum lip scary shrink bird had told me in the room alone she wanted to use some old fashioned therapy where you were drugged loads and like hypnotised or something."

I knew what comedy girl was referring to. I didn't need to acknowledge it though. Her eyes spoke her concern.

"I was shitting myself being ushered into one of the side rooms on the ward. I didn't want to go. I didn't want to stay. Mum and my sister were also professing their objections. Little boy bitch doctor said nothing still. My sister stared at his trouser zipper. It made him blush and shuffle awkwardly so...she did it more. I continued to say I was ok and that I didn't need to be here. Some of the nurses had moved forward to the corridor. They were headed by the one nurse who wasn't my favourite and me not hers. I looked, she stared. I knew what they were limbering up for, like vultures waiting to pounce. I was frightened. Really frightened. Plum lip shrink called for the nurses to restrain me. I was stood still not trying to move but again she called the attack order. The head nurse (the not my favourite one) put her arms out each side. She would not allow her colleagues to go forward. Plum lips became increasingly frustrated with this. She grabbed my arm and shouted restrain her. I had no idea what was going on. No one was moving. The nurse leader one said "No, know one is going to restrain her. There is nothing wrong with her. She doesn't need to be here." Shrink shouted, she is ill, sick, she is dangerous. Head nurse then calmly said "I know this person, I have nursed her and she is not ill.""

Comedy girl moved forward on her seat. She continued "I wasn't following this at all. All I knew was I was full up of fear. And at last somebody was on my side. My mum and sister shouted in unison for me to run."

"and did you?" I couldn't help but ask

"Hell yes I ran, I ran so fast and for so long. I ran in case they were chasing me, then I ran in case the police were coming for me then I ran cos I didn't know what else to do. My mind was going crazy thinking I was going to be found and dragged back. That she was going to be allowed to continue pumping me full up of drugs. I didn't know where to go. I left my car in the car park in case they traced it, or followed it or something equally cop show like. I had no idea what was going to happen and so as you can guess my mind ran wild with horrible endings. I just kept running and as I did so every bit of innocent belief that I held as a kid fell off me. Every bit of trust and simplicity was dragging me down and so I threw it away. I ended up at the young ones place. It was somewhere I thought no one would look. And I hid"

"Shit that sounds awful. Did you hide there all day?" I had understated what I was thinking inside. I was scared for comedy girl.

"Yeah it was fuckin awful. I hid there that day and the next. I hide there three maybe four days. I only came out of the bedroom to pee. I was too scared and as you can guess too paranoid. I thought I was a fugitive."

"How was it sorted or wasn't it" I was making myself cross with the silliness of my questions but I didn't know what else to say. For me it really was the stuff nightmares were made of.

Welcome to My World

"After a few days my uncle rang nurse leader who happened to be the head leader nurse who hadn't clicked well with me. The same one who like a gladiator in waiting had stopped her troops from attacking. She said it was ok. That I wasn't meant to go back and that things would be sorted." I came out of the bedroom but only into the other rooms in the flat. I stayed a while longer. I collected my car in the middle of the night. And for a couple of weeks maybe more I was filled up with fear at every noise, every police man, every person I saw who saw me.

As time elapsed so my fear became less. It never quite left, just became less. Two days before my nursing course started I got a phone call. It was from the nursing school saying there had been a mistake and that I couldn't start the course. I asked why. The woman on the end of the phone was awkwardly searching for words. "Well we have had a letter."

"From who?" I asked. "From the doctor treating you" she replied. "We are unable to accept you anymore." With that she put down the phone. I didn't need any more information. I knew who she was referring to. I'd given up my job ready for the course and now all of a sudden everything felt lost."

"What do you mean?" I questioned. "Had the scary plum lip shrink written to them?"

"Yes" she replied. "It wasn't until later I found out what she had written in detail. She had really gone for it though. I hated her for it, for what she was and what she had done to me. I truly did. I was scared though. Scared to fight back in case she got me locked up in the Looney bin."

In the same week my mum and dad had received a call from some big wig lawyers wanting to meet and discuss with everyone the goings on at the hospital. Mum and Dad said ok although they didn't really know what was meant by this. I went round to see them to, my sister was also there and we sat and listened. It seemed that plum lip shrink had been up to no good with a number of people. The list of her wrong doings was extensive and I had to feel grateful for, in comparison, my relatively lucky escape. They asked me questions. I got upset. They asked if I wanted to sue her or something like that. I didn't want to. I didn't want to recount what had happened to anyone. I was scared. I just wanted to forget about it all. It felt like it was something I watched on the telly. Not real life, not me.
I spoke to them about the nursing course. They said something would be done. I didn't believe them. I was to scared to go to court. The big wig rounded tummy lawyers said that they had enough 'evidence' without my contribution but I would not be compensated. I didn't care.

The next few weeks moved so fast. I was asked to go to two independent evaluations of my mental health by proper in charge shrinks. It was to do with the nursing course because of what plum Lip Shrink had wrote. The Beer Belly big wig lawyers had it all arranged. When I went, the doctors showed me the letters she had written to the nursing people. It was shocking and I knew then immediately why I had been rejected. The list of illnesses was lengthy and of course there was medication to match. Now I understand....then I didn't. The evaluations were ok, questions filled up the time. I was scared of going because now I was scared of everything even remotely linked to doctors or hospitals or anything where a name is put to something. Like being labelled with something…or nothing at all. There was so much power stuck to it.

The doctors found me to be ok, absolutely ok, a little generous I felt but I wasn't hanging about to argue. They contacted the nursing school and I was offered a place in the next intake, only a few months away. I was also offered a job at the sister hospital in the next town for the four months leading up to that time. This was as an apology for what had happened. The little bit of fight left in me rejected that offer. I said I was able to get my own job, not be given one like a charity case. I never stopped believing in myself.

Inside I knew I would not be strong enough to start the nursing course in a few months. My spirit had been crushed a little bit."

Comedy story girl looked up at me. She was smiling.
"What happened to the lipstick shrink?" I asked.
"Well her case went to court, I think it did anyway, there was plenty to choose from in her cruel list of unnecessary interventions. She was found to be in the wrong. (Ya think!) Her doctors licence thing was taken away and she wasn't allowed to be a shrink doctor here any more. I think she returned to her home country. I think but I don't care as long as she never is near me. Maybe it was all done on the quiet. That happens sometimes. I don't know what else happen. I didn't want to listen. She had so much power and had abused every bit of it. She had tried to screw up my world and my dreams. She screwed a lot of people over; she made a lot of people really quite poorly. She was sick….so very sick, I don't know if she was ill though?.

And me, I was left with this big medicine mountain to climb. All these pills doing goodness knows what to my body. My doctor was cool. He let me take control of slowly, very slowly, stopping them all. I would talk to him about what I was doing, I hid nothing but he let me do it my way. I learnt everything I needed to about drugs, everything and then some. I made sure I was fully aware of the dos of the don'ts and of the stuff that was going on and why. Sometimes I stopped something a bit quick and had to adjust it for a while. Sometimes I felt more shit for a while but I knew it would be ok. Sometimes the pills worked against each other. As long as I had control all of the shitty things I felt would be worth it. I was lucky to get the chance to rebuild something. Others had not been so lucky, they were too damaged.

Chapter Ten

From that first day of stopping to the last pill I took was years. I wasn't perfect. Like I said before I'd always been a bit different. I thought about things in a different way, understood things differently. I got the wrong end of the stick sometimes. It didn't make me ill though. At school people who looked at me, but never saw who I was, thought I was slow. Or maybe full of naughtiness. I just learnt differently and no amount of medicine would ever mend that. What always amazes me is that I sometimes have trouble to explain stuff but I never once had a problem saying the most inappropriate or ridiculous things in the world. Like the time just after New Year I had to go to the doctors. I had a bit of a lump. I walked in bold as brass. Sat on the bed/couch thing, looked directly at the doctor and said to him "Hi, I've come to show you my boobs because I didn't send you a Christmas card." You see there was never a need to say it. Let alone so eloquently. I do it all the time.

So anyway, I was saying some of the bits of me got a little bit of a battering when I was all drugged up.   It might only be coincidence that they don't work as well now as they used to. I don't think about it anymore. I don't want to. But anyway I did it. I was so determined to make good of what had happened. To work hard and to over come anything that got in my way. No body was ever going to get close enough to hurt me again. It was just the way I was. Lipstick shrink had tried to steal my dreams.   Lipstick shrink had played dirty but I won."

I had to ask the seemingly obvious question because I wanted to hear Comedy girls answer "Why did you start drinking, you know…that much?

She looked "if you had of asked me then, when I first began, I probably would have said...because I could. But now I think it was much simpler than that. I spent all my time trying to learn the 'rules', the way things should and shouldn't be. I tried to learn at home but then there, what was ok one day was not the next. If you said sorry it made something better but then sometimes you had to say it four times, sometimes eight times, and sometimes it didn't matter how many times you said it. The rules kept on changing. When I used to drink, get drunk or get stoned I broke all the rules. Everything relaxed. My want to understand became a seat for my need to be free. My words that got stuck sailed neatly through the optics. It just made sense. Do you get me?"

Comedy girl stopped talking; she was done with her story. I looked out of the window. How crazy life is. I began to think of my nurse training. How I had got myself a job at 18. I smiled as I remembered. In the interview the woman had asked about my health. I had given her a full run down of my medical past and she had let me. She then said...I actually meant your back! I was always one for giving a little extra on the question answer thing. You see in my world everything is right or wrong, good or bad. I used to need something to help cope with the stuff that didn't fit in.

My nurse training wasn't until much later but I was so proud of what I had achieved. Before then I had a couple of little naughties in my early twenties. A couple of shall we call them 'not so sober' moments...as good as they ever could be, just to see what being really wasted was like. I remember a night in Paris. It was in a '24' hour Karaoke bar. I was with my friend Nat and we'd gone on a little away break. Brook did not belong to the bar; she was from America, in Paris on business. She had dragged her 'not so trendy' colleague out with her. He sat with no expression all night…and it was. Brook instantly became my new best friend. The three of us, me, Nat and my new best friend Brook, discovered an obvious talent that night that had laid dormant forever before. Thankfully at 6.30am the following morning we put that talent back to bed. That's as much as you're getting. Some stories stay private.

So then the nurse training. During which time I met a lovely nurse called Abby. A little part of me wondered if it was the very same comedy girl Abby…that would be cool I liked her a lot. I still see her sometimes where I work and as we pass in the corridor we exchange a silent smile that says so many words.

Then I went on to train to be an instructor in restraining patients. That was a weird thing. Really wanted to do that but then there was one day it got kind of crazy. I had to do training with a couple of people I used to know, years before they didn't recognise me but then that happens with age. They were the kind who always took control in restraints. It was surreal, it put me off a bit. Abby did the training with me too, she said she liked the way I did it. It made me feel proud inside.

This one time on the training I was with a really good group. They were funny. One of the nurses worked nights. She had done for twenty something years I think she said. I'd seen her around the place a few times before. We always said hello. It was like when you know each other that sort of feel. After the group went home I found a note on my desk. It was from the night nurse lady and it read "You made it". It made me smile.

A few months ago I had to go on to a ward to help with an assessment. I do that sometimes in my job. One of the other patients on the ward passed me in the corridor, then a few seconds later passed me again, and again and I looked at her, and the lady, Gwen looked right back at me. She said nothing and then walked away. She remembered forever ago.

I love being a nurse. Every day made me feel strong and proud and lucky to have the chance. I love learning new stuff. It's worth every second it takes. I've stopped trying to find the answers for the things I can't change. Some things are just that little bit different in me. I don't want it to have a name because I have a name.

Id whistle-stop toured my journey to now because there is so much that is good, it's a whole different story. So now when someone asks me what I'm motivated by, to work hard and to keep on learning I have the words. I always knew the reasons and they are the best kind. I believe in my dreams.

I thought for a minute...Im a nurse, comedy girl was a patient. I do restraint, she was restrained. I can prescribe, she was prescribed. I use the Mental Health Act, she was detained. But this was years ago I reckon. It wouldn't happen now. I questioned myself and then comedy girl replied....."Not on my shift!". I smiled.

Id loved listening to my coffee companion, to her adventures. I'd learnt stuff and she had made me laugh. I felt like we were old friends and in some ways a little bit similar. I looked back from the window to express my pleasure and thank her for sharing with me. She wasn't there. No bags, no Bart Simpson earmuffs. No sign of her at all. On the table were my empty latte cups and then next to them three full ones all very cold. I again checked around the coffee house with my eyes shut just to see if comedy girl was around but I knew she wouldn't be. I reckon she was hiding.

I suppose I was delaying the inevitable in which ever way I could....that being the coffee house bar stool dismount. I flung my satchel over my shoulder; it caught one of the full cups of coffee and knocked it flying. My new top wore most of it but I sprang up trying to avoid the total amount landing on me like a poor excuse for Tie dye fashion. As I did so my 'across the shoulder' satchel hooked its self under the seat of the stool. This created a barrier to my spring up movement and I was suddenly not going quite where I thought I would be. As the cosmopolitan window bar stool lost its balance so did I. We together went crashing to the floor and I was off. Possibly, the dismount needed a little more work. I paused for a moment and then, I comedy waved at the coffee house audience as I left. And so another adventure begins... Welcome to my world.

Lightning Source UK Ltd.
Milton Keynes UK
26 November 2010

163515UK00001B/10/P